PRAKASH N. DESAI is a professor of clinical psychiatry at the University of Illinois at Chicago and chief of psychiatric service at the VA West Side Medical Center in Chicago. He has also held appointment on the Committee of South Asian Studies of the University of Chicago.

D0907090

Health and Medicine
in the Hindu Tradition

Health/Medicine and the Faith Traditions

Edited by James P. Wind

Health/Medicine and the Faith Traditions
explores the ways in which major religions
relate to the questions of human well-being.
It issues from Project Ten, an interfaith program
of The Park Ridge Center for the Study of
Health, Faith, and Ethics.

Barbara Hofmaier, Publications Coordinator

The Park Ridge Center
is part of the Lutheran General Health Care System.

The Park Ridge Center
676 N. St. Clair, Suite 450
Chicago, Illinois 60611

Health and Medicine in the Hindu Tradition

CONTINUITY AND COHESION

Prakash N. Desai

Crossroad · New York

1989

The Crossroad Publishing Company
370 Lexington Avenue, New York, N.Y. 10017

Printed in the United States of America

Library of Congress Cataloging-in-Publication Data

Desai, Prakash N.
   Health and medicine in the Hindu tradition : continuity and
cohesion / Prakash N. Desai.
      p.   cm. — (Health / medicine and the faith traditions)
   Bibliography: p.
   Includes index.
   ISBN 0-8245-0914-5
   1. Medicine, Ayurvedic.   I. Title.   II. Series.
   [DNLM: 1. Health. 2. Medicine, Ayurvedic.   WB 50.1 D442h]
R605.D46   1989
615.5'3—dc20
DNLM/DLC
for Library of Congress   89-10032
                                                            CIP

R
605
.D46
1989

To the memory of my father,
Navinkant Kesarlal Desai (1910–1987).
He gave me permission to wrestle with his tradition.

Contents

Foreword

So small has our world become that it seems a short reach to quote a Ganda saying from Africa to preface an Indian author's book on health for a largely North American readership. The Ganda say, "He who never visits thinks his mother is the only cook."

Dr. Prakash N. Desai has been destined to spend much of his life far from the spiritual kitchen of his mother's home cooking. To inhabit that room and then to carry with him its mental furnishings and appliances as he entered the West, the medical profession, and the complex world of psychiatry has forced him to come to terms with many figurative menus and cuisines.

I mention his problem and adventure because it helps prepare the reader for the problems and adventures that beckon for attention in the pages that follow. Although his book will reach India, where its market seems limitless—seven out of ten among India's 700 millions practice some form of Hinduism—it has two primary audiences in North America, and readers in each will share some measure of the unfamiliarity about which Dr. Desai writes.

First are the several hundred thousand Americans who come from India or other nations where Hinduism is a strong presence and who, with Desai, have to relate—a favorite word for the author and for Hinduism—tastes inherited from mother's kitchen and father's house to very different influences wherever they turn in America. It is hard to imagine that any of them would not profit from an encounter with the sage and empathic guide who has written this book of explanations.

The book's second audience is among the several million Americans who describe themselves as secular, Christian, Jewish, or "other" than Hindu. They, too, have tastes developed in particular kitchens, and here they have the opportunity to come to terms with those nurtured in another pantry that still often seems far away. The distance narrows constantly, however. The world of Hinduism has grown near for Americans seeking healing and wholeness. This book touches on both how immediate are the gifts of x: Health and Medicine in the Hindu Tradition

Hinduism and how difficult they are to understand, to say nothing of appropriate, out of context. *Health and Medicine in the Hindu Tradition* provides
that context.

When I first read this manuscript I noticed, as a reasonably typical
Western reader, how often I was stumbling upon semifamiliar concepts over
which I had often stumbled before. This time I had Prakash Desai's hand to
guide me over the literary terrain. Turn a page and suddenly you find the
"guru" explained. Thirty years ago few non-Hindu Americans had heard the
word; now it belongs to the suburban vocabulary. The American couple
hurries after work to the neighborhood YMCA to practice yoga. Yoga can
often appear to be a market item, a commodity in the catalog of techniques.
On these pages suddenly one meets it in its context, where it appears in a
different light.

I could cite scores of other references to the way Hindu approaches
impinge upon the Westerner's world. She turns on television or pages
through a magazine and comes across "reincarnation," offered as still another
product for the market; any well-educated person is expected to know about
this concept, and any spiritually mobile person is told how to appropriate it.
But in the Hindu tradition the concepts of reincarnation are webbed into a
fabric of meanings whose contexts one needs if they are to make sense.

From both sets of kitchens, then, from both spiritual worlds, there are
offers of startling, sometimes threatening, and often promising engagements.
Such engagements in this book appear accessible and even urgent. They are
also likely to produce a side effect. The meeting of these worlds in the minds
of the Desais of the world (people of Hindu tradition in the West) and in the
minds of his readers (mostly people of the West) will cause reappraisals of the
meanings and practices brought from both worlds. Dr. Desai suggests that
this process is going on when he dedicates this book to his father, who
allowed him to "wrestle" with the tradition.

In the tradition influenced by the Bible, wrestling is also an appropriate
metaphor. Jacob, to be called Israel, "wrestles" with an angel through a long
night. Job, in his suffering, figuratively wrestles with the God who leaves him
asking "Why?" about that suffering. But in the Hindu tradition, which with
its myriad scriptures, ideas, and prescriptions invites and even demands
wrestling, as in Jewish and Christian worlds, such wrestling can produce
human good.

The encounter, from the first word, is not easy for most people. The Desai
who enters medical school comes across a world where most of the meanings
simply exclude reference to "god" or "gods." You won't find the reference to
gods in the textbooks. Yet the same Desai moves in a Jewish-Christian

culture where "God," a single God, appears everywhere, from coinage to common speech. The response to a single God, monotheism, is a bewildering reality to someone bred in Hinduism, where many gods form the surrounding and interior spiritual realities.

Conversely, Westerners who seek benefits from Hindu concepts and techniques—and millions of Americans are in that number—find that many of these come attached to ideas both alienating and alluring. The profusion of gods, the boundlessness of scriptures (where is the canon?), the rituals and practices are at first bewildering. This book may reduce the scale of bewilderments, puzzlements, and occasions for stumbling, but along the way there is "wrestling."

To take but one example: a quarter century before this book was written, Christian America experienced a voguish, short-lived sensation called "the death of God theology." I recall one evening hearing a representative of that school describe the benefits of secularity. His concluding remarks turned to the Hindu world as the best example of the overly spiritual, superreligious complex. He detailed Western ideas of hygiene, depicting the ways modern medicine brought health to millions. Then he described how in India Hinduism impelled millions to engage in ritual bathing, in rivers polluted with human feces and the refuse of cities above the bathing site. Of course, such bathing killed; it could not heal. So our theologian announced that it was his mission, in the post-God world, to do what he could to eliminate misery by eliminating religion and, in this case, working against Hindu practice. "I'd tell the bathers to stay home, to avoid the river, to remain healthy. But, what the hell, I guess I'm just too secular."

I have a hunch that Dr. Desai would have trouble joining some of his kin jumping into that river and that the wrestling referred to in his dedication extends to many other such practices. Now and then we get glimpses of how the Hindu tradition is in transition in his life, as in so many. He was taught how to depart from the tradition, which means in part how to segregate religion from the rest of life. His father had a wholistic approach, one that produced for him the "continuity and cohesion" promised in the subtitle of this book. We read that this exasperated father one day blurted, "What you young people with newfangled ideas call hygiene, we of the older generation call religion."

Religion, by whatever name it is called, envelops the classical Hindu and goes along with his or her children as they travel and taste other ways. That reality is evident on every page of this book about a form of wrestling designed to promote well-being. *Health and Medicine in the Hindu Tradition* will be an aid to those who are at ease in classical Hinduism but who must make sense of the world of "hygiene" of a different sort. It will be another kind of aid to those of Desai's generation and dislocated ways who live inside a non-Hindu culture. But I suspect its greatest gift is a set of understandings and instruments that will make the Hindu ways of conceiving life and experiencing coherence and health more comprehensible and available to those who have never been near the Hindu tradition. Even the act of rejecting most of these ways can be more informed and therapeutic than would rejection merely because of ignorance. People can grow strong through the act of wrestling. This book brings strength and can impart strength.

Martin E. Marty

Acknowledgments

I was propelled very early on the journey that has led me to the writing of this book. One person has influenced my growth and direction more than any other: Raojibhai Patel ('Mota,' the elder, as those of us close to him endearingly call him). To say that Mota introduced me to Western thought would be an understatement. He opened my mind and instilled a spirit of free inquiry in me. A teacher of mathematics at Baroda University, Mota led a small group in discussions on a wide range of issues. We called our group the Renaissance Club, because we grasped the zest of the Renaissance from him.

My first paper on a psychological interpretation of the ancient texts was written in collaboration with Alfred Collins, who took the lead in impressing upon me their polyvalent meanings. Dhirubhai Sheth at the Center for the Study of Developing Societies in Delhi emphasized constantly at our meetings, in both India and the United States, that India must be understood on its own terms. He made me aware of a broad range of issues, from the herbal cure of constipation to the significance of the ancient Vedas to modern physicists.

I am indebted to many others who have helped me bring this work to completion. Patrick R. Staunton, chair of the Department of Psychiatry at Lutheran General Hospital, first encouraged me to undertake this work. He impressed on me that a physician living in the West might be the right person to write a book on the Hindu tradition. I owe him a debt of gratitude for his faith in me. When the work faltered, James Wind of the Park Ridge Center pressed me on. His reading of my initial draft and valuable suggestions helped in my reorganization of the book. I thank Lester H. Rudy, former chair of the Department of Psychiatry, University of Illinois at Chicago, for his continuous support of my work. June McDaniel provided scholarly editorial assistance and also rich background research. Rajiv Desai served as my sounding board during the writing phase and later went over the manuscript to remove odd and Indian English constructions. Mary

Wolska helped me with her tireless and painstaking typing of the manuscript.

I also want to thank the Park Ridge Center for its support of the research necessary in the preparation of this work.

Finally, Dhawal Mehta, now Director of the B. K. School of Management of Gujarat University, has been an intellectual companion from my boyhood. There is no way that I can tease out his contribution to my developed thinking.

·1·
Prologue: A Pilgrimage Begun

I was introduced to the dilemmas of medical ethics early in my training as a physician in the mid-1950s. Today as I ponder the problems of faith and tradition in relation to health and medicine, some memories from that time force themselves on me.

As a first-year student at Baroda Medical College in India, in a dissection hall reeking with formaldehyde, I was shaken at the sight of a cadaver. I could not help dwelling on images of the man "when warm blood flowed through his veins." I wondered about his family and friends, who somehow had neglected to claim him. (It is rare for an Indian to donate his body for research; only an unclaimed body at the morgue or in the streets ends up on a dissection table.) The Hindu tradition, of which I was a part, had apparently disowned this man. As a child I had learned that the performance of specific rituals marking the passage from one stage of life to another was a Hindu imperative. The last rite of cremation assured passage to another world, the world of ancestors, with whom one would be at home. Yet here in the world of medicine I had to work on a corpse that had not been claimed and cremated. I wonder now how this experience is woven into my search for the meanings of my traditions.

Later on, the joys of caring and curing replaced my brooding and sustained me through medical school. My decision to become a psychiatrist offered me some distance from the disease and death that surrounded me. Possession of a stethoscope had brought unexpected pleasure, and so had delivering babies. But the discovery of hidden dimensions of the psyche came to dominate my mental world. The psychology of illness and the illness of the psyche seemed to be the most subtly articulated pains. A friend introduced me to Freud, and that sealed my fate.

Toward the end of my apprenticeship, another event brought me face-to-face with the tensions between faith and medicine. I was working as an intern in a small-town hospital. About the third day of my tour of duty, I was called in the night to attend to a dying man. I learned immediately that the man had actually died, that this was known to the nursing staff and the

1

family, and that I had been called in only to certify the death. This act of pronouncing a man dead seemed an awesome responsibility. All the years in medical school had not prepared me for it. There were no courses, discussions, or counseling sessions about death. It was always assumed that medicine was a fight against death and disease. We were filled with a sense of magical power, a faith in science, which brought people back from the brink of death. We had a mission, and we carried out the mission with euphoria. As new converts to this faith, we thought we had almost achieved mastery over suffering. I had encountered death before, but never had the reality struck home so poignantly. It occurred to me that this conspiracy to have me declare a person dead was society's way of humbling me, making me accept defeat as a healer.

My next encounter with death was even more traumatic. By then most of my teachers and colleagues knew that I had set my sights on psychiatry. As a student and an intern, I was often pushed to the front to deal with a difficult patient or his family. This time, again in that small-town hospital, I was asked to speak to the parents of a young boy who had been brought to the hospital from a nearby village. The boy was acutely ill and diagnosed as having intussusception, a condition in which one part of the intestine rides over an adjoining part, producing an obstruction. He was gravely ill and would need immediate surgery. When the surgeon explained all this to the boy's parents, the father decided that the boy was going to die anyway, and he refused surgery. The father explained to me that he wanted the boy to die in his arms and in his own home. The father's refusal had prompted the surgeon to assign me the task of "using psychology" to persuade the father to let the surgeons operate and avert what was otherwise certain death. The sad and tearful father yielded to my persistent pleading "to give the boy a chance." I succeeded but not for long. The patient died on the table. I was now asked to announce the boy's death to the family. I was completely deflated. Even today, as I recall the events of that day, I find the sad and accusing eyes of that father staring at me. A chill passes through my body, and yet I still am not sure how I should have acted. Most disturbing about my behavior, I now realize, was my arrogant belief in the miracles of modern medicine. This belief prompted me to brush aside the beliefs of that family as ignorance and backwardness. But should not a physician be filled with certainty, to be able to infuse hope into his patients? Is not such a conviction also part of the healing potion a physician must mix with his ministration? Similar dramas are played out every day on many hospital wards, where physicians make heroic efforts and do "everything" in defiance of death. Yet the father's eyes make easy answers impossible.

Coming to the United States later to specialize in psychiatry, I realized the significance of the culturally conditioned feelings, thoughts, and relationships that bear on conflicts and their resolution and on psychological suffering and its alleviation. The scientific spirit seeks universal application of discoveries about the human mind, based on the idea that ultimately biology is the basis of behavior. As my American patients taught me about the values that governed their deepest assumptions, my Indian patients raised questions in my mind and cast doubt on my newly acquired understandings of their behaviors. Their world was driven by conflicts and needs and also by their assumptions about being and becoming. The force of tradition was manifest in every self-presentation. It gradually dawned on me that help-seeking behaviors and the responses of the help-giving system were grounded in a tradition. I could then see that the faith traditions configured in what we call religion embodied the basic conceptions and experiences of humanity: pains, dilemmas, ambitions, and the desires in which a person's relationships are wrapped.

My attention was thus directed to an understanding of the cultural and traditional differences between the West and the East, particularly the United States and India. I came to realize that as an Indian psychiatrist in the United States, I would need to dissect and decipher the meanings of my patients' behaviors in a way that would acknowledge their diverse cultural and religious origins. I thought I had transcended the markings of my tradition, but my interactions with my children exposed the fragility of my sense of emancipation from Hindu tradition. The words of my father, "You will understand when you have your own children," began to haunt me. My most significant discovery on this journey into my personal and collective past is that India does not let go. India hangs on, though miles and years away. I know that India lives within me, and I come upon a piece here and there on many an inward journey. I hang on to my tongue scraper, an object of some curiosity to American friends who have seen this curved metal strip among my toiletries.

The assertions in this book are a story of my pilgrimage *(yatra)* through both my medical and traditional life. I have become reacquainted with some sources of my tradition, but it can be argued that the route I have taken is only one of many available, that when I reach my destination, I will have missed many important shrines and not crossed rivers significant to others. My tradition is my best apology for not being comprehensive. One simply cannot be.

In this personal statement I have been guided by the spirit that seeks to repair the fracture between medicine and tradition. This spirit points to the limitations of modern medicine yet is also aware that traditions have their limits. Faith and science are always bound to be in some degree of tension, and many people adapt to such tensions by compartmentalizing their lives and minds, avoiding a disabling sense of dissonance. They are able to separate their professional lives from their personal lives almost completely. Over the long haul, this strategy becomes injurious to their well-being.

I remember an Indian saying to a Westerner, "You split the psyche from the *soma,* so you have to worry about putting them together. You have to invent psychosomatic medicine. Our tradition has no such problem." The problem in India is rather that science and tradition have never achieved separate and equal status. Hindu attitudes toward body, mind, and environment emphasize confluence rather than differentiation, the object has not quite become separate from the subject,[1] and the Western celebration of mastery over nature has never quite become a value.

An appreciation of the dynamic interplay between the philosophical and religious thought and the evolution of the theory and practice of medicine is the object of this work. In order to place Hindu medical theory and experience in the larger context of life I have stressed the basic concepts of the self, the body, and society from their beginning. To do otherwise is to isolate health and illness in the domain of a medical school curriculum and to ignore the meaning that tradition and culture impart to the experience of suffering or healing, or especially death. Another reason for an elaborate treatment of the Hindu belief systems is to demonstrate the continuities and discontinuities between the ancient and the modern. The enduring character of the Hindu ethos demands that we delve into the minds of the ancients and into the universe of assumptions they constructed to guide their existence. Their search for cohesion and authenticity spilled over naturally into the never quite separated territory of physicians and thus became part of my study. It is my hope that the insights derived from such an inquiry may further an understanding of the tensions of living in India today.

A particular myth from the epic *Ramayana* comes to mind.[2] King Trishanku wanted to ascend to heaven with his body—not an uncommon motif in Hindu yearning—but brahmin priests refused to perform the necessary ceremonial sacrifices. The maverick priest Vishwamitra, nonbrahmin in origin, took on the task with a vengeance. Vishwamitra performed the sacrifice, and Trishanku began his ascent to heaven in his human form. The gods, however, barred his entry, and he was thrown down to earth. Vishwamitra could not allow him to fall, so he was stopped in the middle, neither in heaven nor on earth. The story of Trishanku is often told to illustrate what becomes of people who strive for what is not theirs to achieve, those who defy a natural order. I have often felt like Trishanku, stuck between two cultures. I have undertaken the present task in the hope of resolving the contradictions created within myself and maybe getting back down to earth.

·2·
Historical and Cultural Overview

India with all her charm and variety began to grow upon me more and more, and yet the more I saw of her, the more I realized how very difficult it was for me or for anyone else to grasp the ideas she had embodied. It was not her wide spaces that eluded me, or even her diversity, but some depth of soul which I could not fathom, though I had occasional and tantalizing glimpses of it. She was like some ancient palimpsest on which layer upon layer of thought and reverie had been inscribed, and yet no succeeding layer had completely hidden or erased what had been written previously.

Jawaharlal Nehru, *The Discovery of India*

"We are an ancient civilization," the Hindus proudly declare. With a glow of self-admiration, Hindus point to a long history of civilized life and a culture rich in its discussions of ancient as well as contemporary issues. Parents tell children stories of their ancient forebears in order to impart to them not only a sense of history but also moral lessons to guide their daily actions. Young and old, men and women, recount the tales of their mythologized ancestors to reinforce feelings of continuity and cohesion. The agony of contemporary life is often explained as a result of estrangement from the past. Today's achievements are traced to the store of knowledge and skills (still incompletely appreciated) of the founders of Hindu civilization. In the performance of daily rituals, as well as in meeting the crises of life, people turn to the traditions handed down through centuries.

TRADITION AS PALIMPSEST

Rituals are pervasive in Hindu life. Life begins with rites and ends with them. No domain of life is free from expectations of behavior that are informed by centuries of traditions. Tradition is the organizing principle of

5

Hindu *samsara,* the flow of Hindu life. And Hindu religion is not only a matter of adoration of god or gods: religious life cannot be separated from life itself in its entirety.

Birth and death are accompanied by rituals formulated more than a millennium before the beginning of the Christian era. Well-being and illness are experienced within the context of the traditional understanding of the body, as well as the psychosocial and environmental orbits of the person. Images of gods and goddesses, enshrined as they are in ancient and modern temples, are also to be found on calendars; idols abound in homes as well as in places of work and business. In choosing a mate, scheduling a wedding, or selecting a date for surgery, one consults an astrologer. A surgeon would not operate, nor would a patient wish to be operated on (except for life-threatening emergencies), on a new-moon night, which is considered inauspicious for undertaking any significant activity. Many in India today believe that their country's troubles as an independent republic stem from the fact that the transfer of authority from the British occurred on an astrologically inauspicious night.

The flowing Ganges evokes images of generations before, as the city of Benares, sitting on the bank of this holiest of rivers, echoes lives lived centuries past. Hindus bathe on the *ghats* (steps to the banks) of this river, and they recall their ancestors reverentially and make offerings to their gods. On another *ghat,* half-cremated bodies are offered back to the waters from whence life, Hindus believe, originally arose. Many terminally ill patients come here to pass their remaining days in the hope of a funeral on the bank of the Ganges, the mother of all.

Widows come to this city to lead a holy life until death comes, their lives and fates somewhat relieved by the proximity to gods and immersion in this place of worship. Among the caste Hindus, a widow is believed an ill omen, and none leads so barren a life. In Benares they seek to purify themselves and devote themselves to the single-minded pursuit of holiness, of which they were deprived by the death of their husbands.

An appointed temple agent, for a commensurate fee, will smooth the way through a throng of worshippers at the great temple of the god Shiva, the Lord of Kashi (another name for Benares). There one prays for oneself and one's entire lineage—thus establishing continuity and discharging one's paramount obligation to the spirit of one's dead ancestors. Chanting ancient mantras and offering gifts to the gods, Hindus ask in return for long, healthy, prosperous lives, freedom from disease, and a holy death. The continuity between the past and the present, the ancient and the current, is a truly remarkable feature of the fabric of Hindu India.

The image of a palimpsest is often invoked for the whole national tradition, as Jawaharlal Nehru did or, more recently, as historian of religion Diana Eck does in describing Benares: "The city displays the layering of the Hindu tradition like a palimpsest, an old parchment that has been written upon and imperfectly erased again and again, leaving the old layers partially visible."[1] But there is not one India, not even one Hindu India. The land and its people are not a homogeneous mass. As an archaeologist discovers in excavations strata of earth chronologically arranged and distinct one from the other, so looking at contemporary India one finds a variety of cultural differentiations from different eras and places. A family, a village, and a caste—each can preserve its particular tradition in the midst of political or technological change. Like different parts and tissues of a body—growing, changing, healing, and degenerating at different rates—Hindu communities (and castes and families within them) seem to maintain their own chronologies. The heterogeneity of India, as well as the Hindu tradition, bears marks of the origin and history of the subcontinent. The original inhabitants, successive migrations, invasions, and diffusion of populations over centuries have created a culture with many strata.

Although the words *Hindu* and *Indian* are often used synonymously, this practice can be deceptive. Of the more than 700 million people in India, close to a fifth identify themselves as Muslim, Christian, Sikh, or Jain, or as members of some other religion. One may speak of the Hindu tradition as the dominant tradition and also assert that this tradition has had a major impact on all other traditions in India, but even Hinduism is not just one tradition. More than a fifth of the population consists of the tribals and the so-called untouchables. Most of these people may describe themselves or may be regarded as Hindus, but their actual traditions, gods, rituals, forms of worship, and beliefs about relationship are at significant variance from the dominant brahminic tradition. The Hindu tradition itself has gone through a variety of transformations and bifurcations and has even spawned new religions. This process began when the Aryan people settled in India and continues today. Variations on any theme can always be found. In the words of historian Nirad Chaudhari, "It is as if the historic and living Hinduism was an elaborate cadenza to an unplayed composition, on which the Hindus have been improvising variations in near and distant keys without feeling that they are being unorthodox."[2] A brief review of the sources of these traditions is warranted.

ARYANS AND HARAPPANS

The word *Hindu*—not of Indian origin—is the Persian name of a river known to people of the subcontinent as Sindhu, which now lies mainly in

Pakistan.[3] *Sindhu* became *Hindu* to the Persians and *Indus* to the Greeks, and from *Indus* is derived *India*. The religion of the people who inhabited the fertile plains of this river came to be known as Hindu, and the name was eventually applied to the people themselves by those coming into contact with them (including, of course, their invaders, such as Alexander of Macedon and his troops, who came to northwestern India in 327 B.C.E.).

The inhabitants of the subcontinent themselves knew of no such people or religion. The writers of the earliest religious literature called themselves Aryans, meaning "the noble"; they called their religion *sanatana dharma*, or eternal religion. Another term that has also been applied to this body of traditions is *Brahminism*, since the religious elite of the time were brahmins. When the population moved to the south and east, they occupied a triangular area—the plains bounded by the Indus and Ganges rivers. A part of the area between the rivers Ganges and Jamuna was known to the people of the plains as Aryavarta, the land of the Aryans. The original stratum of Hindu tradition is the outgrowth of the religious philosophy of these people.

Before the Aryans came to India, the Indus valley was populated by a people of different racial origin. Their culture spread from northwestern India to the lower reaches of Rajasthan and upper Gujarat in western India. The Indus Valley civilization and the later Harappan city culture are known to us mainly through archaeological remains.[4] The civilization of the people of the Indus Valley stretches far into antiquity, perhaps as far as 10,000 B.C.E. Communities became settled as agriculture flourished. These village communities later built the cities of Harappa and Mohenjo-daro, known for their advanced plumbing and architecture. They built fortified cities on exactly the same sites in identical fashion after each successive flooding, a mark of their conservatism.[5] Their elaborate bathhouses lead one to speculate whether the later emphasis in Hindu India on bathing is a gift of the Harappan people.

Modern sanitation in India is very different from the older Harappan system which had elaborate drains and sewers built under the streets leading to soak-pits. These attest to their concern about health and sanitation, as do their public bathhouses. Of the many buildings excavated, none appears large enough to suggest a temple.[6] We know from their seals and terra-cotta figures that animals, especially the bull, were an important part of their lives. Statuettes of women, mostly naked and with intricate headdresses, perhaps represented mother-goddesses, and a proto-Shiva can be constructed from an ithyphallic figure sitting in a yoga position surrounded by beasts. This has led to the speculation that the Hindu god Shiva, as well as yoga (the meditative and health-related Hindu practice most closely associated with Shiva as arch-yogin), are also derived from the Harappans.

From about 2000 to 1500 B.C.E., the invading Aryans overwhelmed the Harappans, first displacing them and later assimilating their culture. We may conclude from the literature of these Indians that they were fair-skinned, while the original inhabitants were dark-skinned. The Aryan victors considered the native inhabitants to be servile, enslaved, and inferior, but most important, they were non-Aryan. The superiority of the invaders' war technology, especially their more effective weapons and horse-driven chariots, must have held the edge in battle. The major god of these people, Indra, is also known as Purundar, destroyer of the fortified city Pur. These Aryans were nomads: cattle breeders and meat eaters in search of a home which they found in India. This era of Indian history, although an object of enormous scholarly exploration, remains obscure because of the lack of any written materials.

India is as much a land of immigrants as the North American continent. Over a period of several thousand years, people traveled in caravans through the northwestern Himalayan mountain passes or on ships to the vast coastal peninsula. Among these groups of immigrants, only the Aryans so overwhelmed the settled inhabitants. Hence the pervasive and lasting impact of these people, later called Hindus. The main sources of our knowledge of this era are the Vedas, the earliest surviving literature of the Hindus, which were composed between 1500 and 1000 B.C.E. and were committed to memory. The first traces of Hindu medicine, as we shall see, are in the Vedic compendia.

HISTORY AND MEMORY

The Hindus have a sense of history very different from that of Westerners. A tradition of assigning specific dates is absent in early India; it only becomes available through the journals of Greek, Persian, and Chinese visitors. Dating later becomes manifest in the Indian Islamic tradition. Ashis Nandy, a scholar expert in political and cultural psychology, argues that the Indian culture was not ahistorical but approached history via three mediators. The first group were the minstrels, or *charons*. Wandering individually or in groups, they sang of past events or of the heroic acts of men, "giving meaning to the present by projecting its rough realities into a mythologized past." The second group of mediators were genealogists and chroniclers, who constructed "formal generational continuity." The third were the court historians, who created "larger-than-life subjects out of the mortals who were their masters and patrons." All three approaches were "deeply embedded in an orientation to the past which reduces or elevates each social reality to a psychologically significant myth."[7]

This typology tells us how Indians use history. What it does not explicitly convey is the intense Hindu preoccupation with the past. *Itihas,* "it happened thus," is intimately relevant to how we do things now. For a Hindu, it is not that "those who forget their history are bound to repeat it"; the Hindu ethos demands that you remember your history and *insists* that you repeat it. Thus, when Hindus glow with pride declaring that theirs is an ancient civilization, the emotion is sincere and profound. They speak of their ancestors of centuries past with a feeling of immediacy and carry the name of their *gotra,* the lineage which dictates specific transactions and forbids others. These forefathers are enshrined in the collective memory through daily observances and are celebrated as the founders of a great tradition. The essential knowledge about the human condition that these mythologized heroes of Hindu faith have taught, contemporary Hindus insist, has helped preserve the tradition in its pristine form.

For Hindus history is a lived-in reality. The survival of major treatises for centuries, written down perhaps only after the development of the Brahmi script (considered to have been finished in about 300 B.C.E.), attests to the emphasis placed on memory—remembering the past and interpreting it to serve the present.[8] This gives to the Hindu culture both a paleocentric and mythopoetic character.

Hindus revere the past, but not only in a religious sense; the past is looked to also for inspiration and prescription of social and personal conduct. The ancient Vedic literature, the later epics, and the medieval tales of the past (*puranas*) illustrate through mythmaking the essential relationships between humans and between humans and institutions. Whether in a family or a classroom, in politics or the workplace, ancient heroes and their deeds are recalled, and the present compared with the past. In the process, old myths change and new ones are generated. Unknown facts are filled in, and the accounts become richer as they pass from mouth to mouth and generation to generation. As every Indian will say, "Don't confuse me with facts; the ones I don't know, I will make up." To complete stories and leave no loose threads is an art form; this can be clearly seen in Indian cinema, where little is left implicit.

This attitude has resulted in flexible rules of ethical and moral conduct. Although Hindus recall their early past to guide them in their actions, the narrative of the conduct of their ancestors is not fixed. With the generation of new myths, the heroes of the legends are given new forms, and stories are adapted to the needs of the present. Different versions of ancient texts exist, and different texts always tell slightly altered accounts of particular events. This constant accommodation gives the Hindus their amazing diversity yet keeps them in the fold.

MEDICAL TRADITION AND FAITH

A way of looking at this diversity is provided by the suggestion that God recedes into the background. God is present, like the Indian drone, the instrument that accompanies all musical recitals. But social strictures seem at times to have greater influence on ordinary conduct than do the religious paths chosen by any member. One can become an "outcaste" by crossing some inviolable social boundary, but one cannot cease to be a Hindu by choosing a different form of worship.

The vast spaces of the subcontinent and the geographic immobility of most Indians have generated separate languages, sufficiently distinct to be mutually incomprehensible. The same separation applies in such areas as custom, food, and ritual. Perhaps herein lies the secret of the survival of the Hindu tradition. Accumulating various interpretations of reality, Hindus arrive at a vision of the good life determined by adaptation and accommodation to prevailing conditions. As the subcultures of multiple ethnic groups were being assimilated into a social order, regulation of behavior appears to have been more important than regulation of beliefs. The private lives of the populace were left alone, and in early India few attempts were made at consolidating a social philosophy that would then govern both public and private behavior. The result is a profound conviction that "truth" or self-realization is discovered through many paths, and a simultaneous rejection of absolutes in considerations of personal morality.

One difficulty in speaking about the "faith tradition" as a distinct object of study is that Hinduism is more a tradition than a faith. In the daily practices of Hindus, traditions are faithfully observed. What might be considered an aspect of secular life in the West, Hindus would assert to be a part of their religion—what they eat, for example, or with whom they eat, or who cooks for them. One also finds religious life pervaded with matters considered profane elsewhere, such as couples in sexual congress on the outer walls of a temple, or the sexual intimacies of gods and goddesses. It is difficult to draw clear lines between that which is tradition, handed down from generation to generation, and that which is derived from religious doctrines. Obligations and duties that direct behavior can probably be traced to some idea about human relationships with God, but more often than not the actor attributes the behavior to the force of *pranalika* (originally meaning a channel or a course flowing down from a reservoir) or tradition. No actions can be viewed outside the moral or religious sphere, and a Hindu scholar can always trace the origin of a ritual or a custom to some spiritual imperative or to some Hindu scripture. However, for a layperson, no conscious knowledge of such a command is required nor does it often exist.

For example, most Hindus practice rinsing—amounting to gargling—before and after a meal. Ordinary understanding regards this simply as healthful, but its origin can be traced to an ancient injunction to do so in order to "dress *prana,* the breath."[9] My father once articulated this link in a rather simple way. Arguing about menstruation taboos—against touching a menstruating woman before her ritual bath—he said, "What you young people with newfangled ideas call hygiene, we of the older generation call religion." Other taboos concern birth, marriage, and death. Medical traditions are continuous with religious traditions.

A distinctly identifiable Hindu medical tradition, the Ayurvedic, exists both in theory and in practice—stretching back two millennia over all of India. The theory is inseparably intertwined with the theological and liturgical discourses of the time. As we shall see, the medical texts articulate religious issues, and the religious texts include issues of diagnoses and therapies. Hindu medicine never became divorced from the rest of life's pursuits, especially not from the religious, as medicine did in the West.

Apart from the dominant Ayurvedic tradition, a second medical tradition, *siddha,* has a following in the south of India. The theoretical principles of this system are largely derived from the Ayurvedic tradition, but its emphasis on oxides of metals in therapeutics was influenced by Greek apothecary.

Then there is astrology. The houses of the horoscope represent sectors of life, designated variously as the seats of health, illness, marriage, progeny, and so on. The heavenly bodies also have specific domains, including those of health and well-being. Astrologers are called on to make predictions, which may lead to specific ritual performances or the wearing of certain stones to ward off or alleviate illnesses. An Ayurvedic physician may draw on the horoscope in calculating the treatment of a particular disorder.

One difficulty in demarcating the medical and health concerns of the Hindus is the introduction of medical systems from the West. It is clear that the Greek Hippocratic medical tradition interacted with the later Ayurvedic tradition, as did the Arabic medical tradition (the Unani), especially in the north of India. More recently, allopathy (the Western modern medical tradition)[10] has come to India—along with the influxes of the Portuguese, the French, and the British—and taken its place alongside competing ideologies and health ideals.

All these influences allow for a complex interplay between pragmatic health concerns and help-seeking behaviors of a traditional people. It is again a measure of the assimilative strength of the Hindu tradition that these contradictory systems coexist, often borrowing from each other at the periphery. The receiver of care is hardly concerned with these contradictions. Just as an Indian uses history for his or her immediate ends, the patient chooses his or her healer to match pressing concerns.[11]

SOURCES OF HINDU TRADITION

A vast collection of Hindu literature has been compiled over centuries. The Vedas, from the verb *vid*, "to know," are the repository of ancient knowledge about the Hindus and their experiences. The *Rig Veda*, the earliest of Hindu texts, is usually regarded as having been composed around 1500 B.C.E. It is a compendium of about 1,080 hymns—invocations of the gods who preside over the earthly realms and songs in praise of their power. More imaginative than contemplative, they show poetically the Aryan's awe before nature.

To the religious philosopher Sarvepalli Radhakrishnan the work of the Vedic poets represents the "earliest phase of religious consciousness, where we have not so much the commandments of priests as the outpourings of poetic minds who are struck by the immensity of the universe and the inexhaustible mystery of life."[12] Jawaharlal Nehru, an avowed atheist, was also impressed by these poets: "The Rig-Veda, the first of the Vedas, is probably the earliest book that humanity possesses. In it we find the first outpourings of the human mind, the glow of poetry, the rapture at nature's loveliness and mystery."[13] Hindus return to the Vedas, especially the *Rig Veda*, as a starting point of their civilization.

Later Vedas contained liturgical treatises, meditations, and philosophical commentaries as well as hymns. The liturgical treatises (*brahmanas*) present narrations of ritual, detailing principally the sacrificial work of the priests. In a world where temples had not yet been built and gods had not assumed iconic forms, the performance of the sacrifice involved the propitiation of the Vedic gods and an invitation to them to reside in the ritual fire. The *aranyakas* are the meditations of forest dwellers and are a starting point for the philosophical commentaries known as the Upanishads.

The Upanishads are writings about the inner meaning of life and death, as given by a father or teacher to his most advanced students. The major Upanishads were composed before 500 B.C.E. and were not taught widely or published, but rather passed on orally in secret. They discuss meditation, the true nature of person and world, states of consciousness, and human fulfillment. They were considered as *shruti*, that which was heard and thus revealed, rather than *smriti*, that which is remembered and considered derivative of the Vedas. This latter category includes the *Mahabharata* and

Ramayana epics, and the *dharmashastras*, or law texts. A principal law text is the *Laws of Manu*.

The *Laws of Manu* is a systematization of the Hindu view of society, containing such categories as the four goals of mankind, the four stages of life, and the four castes (*varnas*). It seeks to unify the two opposing religious goals of Hindus: social obligation (*dharma*), and personal liberation (*moksha*). These are located at different stages of life in *Manu*, and can thus coexist, as division of labor coexists in the caste system.

Another major system of works is that of *darshana*, or philosophy. The two systems most relevant to the issues of health and medicine are those of yoga and *samkhya* philosophy. The origins of these philosophies are traced to early Indian thought and practices. Classical yoga is based on the *Yoga Sutra* of Patanjali (second century B.C.E.), which describes methods to bring the yogin's body and mind under the control of his spirit. The goal is control of the modulations of the yogin's mind—the suppression of states of consciousness. This is done by stages—positive and negative moral rules, postures and breath control, disengagement of the senses from worldly things, concentration and meditation, and perfectly balanced consciousness. The goal of Patanjala yoga is isolation (*kaivalya*), in which the person becomes a pure observer, without attachment.

Yoga is based on the *samkhya* system of philosophy, which emphasizes the dissociation of spirit from matter. Its most important text is the *Samkhya Karika* of Isvarakrishna (200 C.E.). According to *samkhya*, the world is real, but it is based on ignorance of the spirit. The spirit is enslaved by its participation in nature, which is eternally changing and disintegrating. Liberation (*moksha*) means an escape from suffering and attachment, a knowledge of one's true situation, and a renunciation of matter in favor of spirit.

Another significant text is the *Bhagavad Gita*, which occurs within the epic *Mahabharata* (400 B.C.E.–400 C.E.) This epic is the story of the great war within the family of the Bharatas, in which relatives fight over succession to the throne. Its most famous segment is the *Gita*, the "Song of God," in which the warrior-prince Arjuna doubts the value of this warfare, and his charioteer (the god Krishna in human form) discusses why Arjuna can and must fight. Within this discussion arise the topics of duty, action, love, spiritual growth, and religious vision. The *Gita* shows the ideal relationship between god and devotee, mentor and pupil.

The Ayurvedic literature also begins in the pre-Christian era and consists of several texts on health and medicine, the three major ones being the *Carakasamhita* (100 C.E.), the *Sushrutasamhita* (200 C.E.), and the *Ashtangahridaya samhita* (700 C.E.). Pain and suffering, illness and its cure, and the conduct of the care giver are the subjects of these treatises, which will be treated in detail in Chapter 7.

Much in Hindu literature deals with the goals of *kama,* love and desire, and *artha,* wealth and power. The most famous *kama* text is probably the *Kamasutra* of Vatsayana, from the third century C.E. It includes such topics as sexuality, courtship and marriage, prostitution, the sixty-four arts, and the life-style of the man-about-town. Other *kama* texts discuss spells, potions, and further variations of sexual relationships. The most famous text on *artha* is probably the *Arthashastra,* which discusses diplomacy, warfare, and politics.

All these works and others are part of the great Sanskritic, or classical, tradition of India. They interact on the local level with folk and village beliefs—in ancestor worship, spirit possession and exorcism, and worship of local deities. These local traditions are sometimes called the "little traditions," and they have affected the interpretations of the texts of the "great tradition."

Anthropologist McKim Marriott describes the processes of mutual penetration between the great tradition and the several local traditions as universalization and parochialization. By universalization he means a process in which aspects of the little traditions are incorporated into the great tradition. This "carrying forward and upward not only of cultural awareness, but also of cultural contents" has significantly altered the Hindu pantheon. Parochialization, he argues, is the reverse process by which aspects of the great tradition are transformed and move downward into the little tradition.[14] Many Hindu festivals are a good example of this process. There are also processes of upward and downward assimilation in Indian medicine, incorporating other medical traditions like the Unani from the Arabs and allopathy from the West. Practitioners of allopathic medicine incorporate in their idiom Ayurvedic ideas of humors and sometimes prescribe Ayurvedic medicines. The Ayurvedic doctors (*vaidyas*) are equally prone to give penicillin injections and vitamin supplements. Indian medicine at the center strives to preserve its purity, while at the periphery (away from the medical schools) an intermixing of tenets and medicaments can be easily observed among practicing family physicians.

The history and development of Hindu thought is as long as it is varied. It is not possible to tease out the antecedents of current practices to locate their origins, nor to establish authorship and dates. The pre-Aryan heritage of India is inextricably mixed with what the later immigrants spawned. In fact, history as the West understands it is irrelevant to Hindus, who shape their lives by the force of tradition and by the mythologies of their ancestors. Without the central defining authority of a prophet, book, or priestly order, the evolution of Hindu civilization took a variable course. This course was further complicated by geographic diffusion and the entry of hitherto unassimilated groups of people. New religions entered; new sects were formed as new ethics and practices emerged. A continuous process of interpenetration of the great tradition with little traditions gave way to local specialization and a way of life that could call upon convenient sources for justification. Yet underneath all these complexities and elasticities lies a fountain-source of conceptions about the self, the body, and the life course. These often unspoken assumptions lend a coherence to Indian life and are responsible for its continuity.

·3·

Samsara: The Stream of Life

He is only an appendage to his germ-plasm, to which he lends his energies, taking in return his toll of pleasure—the mortal vehicle of a (possibly) immortal substance—like the inheritor of an entailed property who is only the temporary holder of the estate.
Sigmund Freud, On Narcissism

The Indian word *samsara*—meaning the life course, all that happens between birth and death—evokes the image of a river. *Samsara,* literally "that which flows well" or "that which flows together," captures the idea of movement in time. The pace is relentless, swift, and not always predictable. It is not only the course of an individual life, for the flowing together represents mergers and partings. *Samsara* is an apt metaphor for the life course: a river descending from mountain springs, turbulent and frothy, coming swollen to the plains, often nourishing and occasionally destructive. It branches and finally loses its identity as it merges with the ocean. The river is a potent symbol around which Hindu life revolves. A place of pilgrimage is a *tirtha,* a place for crossing from this shore of life to the other, where one is free. Both the *yogin* and the devotee *(bhakta),* like the madman, are said to have gone to the far shore.[1]

ORDER AND LAW

Hindu life is defined by the dynamics of movement, exchange, and limits, and follows a pattern governed by natural laws. Winds, heat, and gravity direct the waters, and their transformations are another metaphor for the processes of life. Moisture, clouds, and monsoons rotate through cycles, as do human beings. Orderly transitions and predictable events were concerns in the earliest Hindu thought. An interest in order *(rita)* arose when the nomadic Aryans were settling down in the plains of north India. Celestial events were experienced as following intrinsic laws; the power of the laws of

17

rita made things happen in expectable ways. Hindu philosophers sought inspiration from the order of the cosmos to define their own conduct and to formulate laws for governing behavior. In the *Rig Veda* we read:

> Order and truth were born from heat as it blazed up.
> From that was born night; from that heat was born the bellowing ocean.
> From the bellowing ocean was born the year, that arranges days and nights,
> Ruling over all that blinks its eyes.
> The arranger has set in their proper place the sun and the moon, the sky and the earth, the middle realm of space, and finally the sunlight.[2]

Here the poets fashioned a cosmogony in which order and truth were the first-born. Human beings were connected to their environment by the workings of the same laws. In this early vision, an abstract notion of unseen but always present order provides an anchor of predictability in the sometimes hostile but more often nurturant nature.

The search for order in individual and collective life reflects a yearning for controls. Unruly passions can overwhelm the intellect, while individual interests may subvert and subordinate group cohesion. The loss of *rita* is captured in the lament of a poet of the *Rig Veda*:

> I ask of thee, the ancient one, . . . where is the *rita* of the past gone?
> Who is the new one who holds it? . . . oh gods of the three spheres, where
> is the *rita* of yours gone? Whence again is this absence of *rita (anrita)?* . . .
> Where is the watchfulness of Varuna (the original custodian of *rita*)? And
> hence we are fallen in misery . . . we ask of Varuna, the knower of the path
> and maker of food, and I utter this from my heart: Let the *rita* be born
> anew.[3]

Even today when the rains fail to come over a protracted time, Hindus commission sacrifices invoking their Vedic lore. The Indian word *ritu*, meaning season (winter, summer, and so on) is derived from *rita*, intimately connected with the flow of time.

Retaining the idea of *rita* in human affairs as moral conduct, the idea of *dharma* replaced the notions of order in nature, in individuals, and in society. *Dharma* is not easily translated in English. From the verb *dhru*, meaning to hold, maintain, and sustain, *dharma* sustains a person and holds a people together much as *dhatus* (from the same verb), substances, hold a body together. P. V. Kane, a jurist and a scholar of religion, suggests that the word comes to mean "the privilege, duties and obligations of a man, his standard of conduct as a member of the Aryan community, as a member of one of the castes, as a person in a particular stage of life."[4] *Dharma* thus came to be understood as the Hindu law, and the voluminous literature dealing with the law came to be called the *dharmashastra*, the law books.

The Hindu emphasis on the interiority of the self has caused the tradition to be labeled introspective, but such a characterization of the entirety of Hinduism fails to appreciate Hindu attention to this-worldly affairs. After all, the Hindu quest for self-realization can be realized through adherence to the law. In the evolution of Hindu thought, a connection was sought between person and cosmos. This was established by the performance of the sacrificial ritual and by the orderly organization of personal and social life. This connection was enhanced by rituals and in turn endowed the concept of order with predictability. The spheres of the human and the divine were reciprocally reinforced. The emergence of the Upanishadic introspective tradition around 1000–500 B.C.E. was an attempt to separate the true and unchanging from the false and ephemeral. In a way, this inward-looking philosophy exposed the inability of brahminical Hinduism to bring coherence to both personal life and an increasingly complex social life.

But the introspective tradition of the Upanishads ushered in an era of highly individualistic spiritual pursuit, and it too fell short of the task of helping the masses cope with the uncertainties of a law-governed universe. The geographic diffusion of populations coupled with battles for political hegemony created a demand for a new social ethic. As the *Bhagavad Gita* was to declare a few centuries later, the path of knowledge was arduous and suited only to the religious elite, while the paths of action and devotion were more appropriate for the masses.

The challenge of maintaining personal and social organization in the face of new social realities was taken up by the formulators of the law books. *Dharma* laid down the rules and ordinances for action in all situations. In *dharma* there was a reversion to the idea of natural order *(rita);* but unlike *rita*, which connected human beings to the course of nature, *dharma* connected them also to each other.

The laws that *dharma* embodied were construed as derivations of Vedic commands, but the elaborations went far beyond the speculations of the Vedic poets. The brahmin priests became the interpreters of *dharma*, and the kings the administrators. Interpretations were designated as the remembered word *(smriti)*, and the force of tradition attached to them. In their rigor and meticulous attention to detail, a passion for overinclusiveness emerged. The obligations of each individual according to age, sex, and station in the evolving social matrix were categorized. Always steering away from absolutes, always sensitive to context, the laws allowed qualifications for time, place, and exceptional circumstances. Laws governing conduct in situations of distress *(apaddharma)* set aside the usual principles of conduct. Common usage and local custom facilitated a variable interpretation of the ancient texts and themselves became a source of *dharma.* The proliferation of the law books was a result of somewhat differing traditions of lineages, some tied to particular Vedas and others to multiple centers of power away from the heartland bounded by the Indus and Ganges rivers.

The tasks of keeping the self from falling apart in the everyday world, and preserving that world intact, were the bases of *dharma.* In the Vedic lore gods were not always synonymous with good and therefore were not moral exemplars. The Upanishadic *atman,* the ageless, interior, and unqualified self, common to all beings and things as the inherent *sat* (truth), could not supply the individual with a guide for action particular to him or her. The assertion of *atman* as the only and ultimate true reality, and the categorization of everything else as false, in fact demolished grounds for conduct according to worldly laws.

The "conduct of virtuous men" able to transmit textual knowledge became a source of inspiration for the masses. If the tradition laid down an elaborate code of conduct for the common folk, the heterodoxy of the elite emphasized "that which was pleasing to the self."[5] Thus inner contentment was added, at least for the elite, as a source of *dharma.*[6]

P. V. Kane, whose encyclopedic *History of Dharmasastra* covers the entire literature of the law books written over almost two millennia, divides that literature into three major strands. The first deals with the performance of sacrificial ritual in public life; the second concerns the duties and ritual obligations of the householder; and the third, collectively the *dharmasutra,* describes the rules of popular conduct, law, and custom. These laws, including the *Laws of Manu,* discuss the four aims of life, the four classes of people, the four stages of life, and a number of sacraments marking passages (the *samskaras*). Digests, redactions, commentaries, and redefinitions have been part of the continuous rewriting of the law books to the present day.

Traditions, customs, rituals, beliefs, and laws enunciated in the law books are as alive today as they were when the texts were composed. In contrast to earlier Vedic formulations, which have been incorporated and subsumed into traditional Hindu life and lore, the ideas and practices of the *dharmashastras* are an explicit and integral part of Hindu traditions in their near-original forms. Many scholars suggest that the *dharmashastras* capture the spirit of proper Hinduism and that the older Vedic literature may be regarded as a philosophical backdrop to them.[7] Others bemoan the corruption of the ancient Vedic religion in later Hindu practices.[8]

THE FOUR AIMS OF LIFE

Virtue *(dharma)*, purpose or wealth *(artha)*, and pleasure *(kama)* motivate human actions. For an ordinary human being, the pursuit of self-realization rests in the acceptance of these three ends. Although disagreement prevailed regarding their hierarchical ordering, the *Laws of Manu* concluded that all three were to be equally pursued.[9] The fourth and supreme end of life is *moksha*, release or liberation from the cycle of rebirth.

Dharma, artha, kama, and *moksha* are principles of human action throughout the course of life. To each person the goals of virtue, wealth, and pleasure are assigned according to his or her situation, especially in relation to caste, status, age, and gender. These aims of life not only guide personal action vis-à-vis God but more stringently ordain relationships with other persons. Husband-wife, parent-child, and teacher-pupil relations, kinship networks, and intercaste relations—all require specific transactions. From early childhood one prepares for these mutual obligations in the family network as well as outside it. Mutuality does not presuppose symmetry: an order of hierarchies in relationships is established. Nurturing this sense of place in a child is a mark of good parenting.

Artha is interpreted as both intention and object. It means the pursuit of livelihood not as an end in itself but as necessary for the sustenance of life. Wealth and material well-being do not violate religious obligations, and a life of poverty is neither comfortable nor enhances self-esteem. *Kama*, pleasure-seeking, reflects acceptance of the realities of human nature. *Kama* refers broadly to the affectional aspect of persons through which they bind themselves to each other. From another vantage point, it is also an effort to integrate and regulate passions. The twin dangers of wild expressions of desire and indiscriminate suppression of impulses are acknowledged. *Artha* and *kama* are thus subsumed under *dharma*, but their separate status attests to the here-and-now attitude in Hindu transactions. These are not just another set of duties, they are entitlements within the scope of a moral life. The legitimation of material goals and the fulfillment of desires permit inclusion of such activities within the ethical domain.

Moksha is different. It is otherworldly, an end in itself, a release from the bondage of works and the cycles of birth and rebirth. It aims to go beyond the body, beyond the physical nature, and it connects the search for immortality with the quest for cohesion. *Moksha* stands for freedom from the experiences of pain, old age, and death but also for merger with the original principle of creation. It is the culmination of appropriately conducted *dharma*.[10]

The four ends of Hindu life are incorporated into the medical literature. As the *Carakasamhita,* the sourcebook of Ayurveda, declares, well-being ("a disease-free state") is to be pursued for the attainment of "virtue, wealth and gratification."[11] The authors of the medical texts show rare practical wisdom in their ability to sidestep confrontation with the priestly order. They did this without divorcing the body from intentions and behaviors or well-being from considerations of habits, personality, and relationships.

A long list of good conduct and virtuous behaviors is offered in the *Carakasamhita* without distinctions among physical, psychological, social, and spiritual considerations. Duties include worshipping gods and brahmins, keeping the sacred fire and offering oblations, respecting the teacher, performing the rites for dead ancestors, not telling a lie or desiring the women or property of others, not being critical of others, and not swimming in strong currents.[12]

Desire for long life, desire for wealth, and desire for the other world are the principal motivations of Ayurvedic prescriptions. The desire to live is first, "because on departure of life, everything departs." Next to life, wealth is sought because "there is nothing more sinful than to have a long life without means [of sustenance]."[13] The Ayurvedic text then goes on to present arguments for and against the notion of rebirth. It decides in favor of a theory of rebirth on the basis of authority, recognizing the limitations of perception, inference, and reasoning.

THE FOUR CLASSES

The division of people into four classes or castes is one of the oldest aspects of the Hindu tradition, originating in the creation myth of the *Rig Veda* (see Chapter 4). The four classes were created from different parts of the body of the cosmic giant Purusha and were also differentiated on the basis of skin color. The Vedic myth has continued to shape Indian society to the present day. The original four classes were the brahmins (priests, scholars, and teachers), the *kshatriyas* (rulers and warriors), the *vaishyas* (traders, bankers, and agriculturalists), and the *shudras* (the toilers and menial workers). The untouchables, a later designation, were outside the system and performed the most menial jobs. The modern division of Indian society is into *jatis,* or subcastes, a proliferation of the original divisions, as well as the incorporation of original inhabitants and new immigrants. The increasing and changing stratification of castes attests that neither have these categories been fixed nor has social organization been static.

Debate continues on whether the four classes were hereditary or determined by the qualities and occupations of people. There is hardly any doubt that further subdivisions of the castes were necessitated by mixed marriages. The *Laws of Manu* gives an elaborate list of the categories resulting from such mixtures, which are seen as posing danger to society and threatening the loss of status and occupation.[14] Rules for the exchange of cooked food were also well-established, including prohibitions against receiving cooked food from physicians and surgeons, people in low occupations and without virtue, and those with undesirable physical or psychological qualities.[15]

The caste system raises a significant question for the present undertaking (and for any study of the contemporary Indian sociopolitical situation): does the social hierarchy assume inherent and substantive differences among people? The answer, unfortunately, is yes. The castes were created unequal by the logic of the body parts of Purusha, the cosmic giant from whom they arose. Besides the laws for exchanges of food, a system of making marriages only between people of similar "virtue" (based on caste, racial stock, and color distinctions) and the *guna* theory of qualitative differences among people came to determine what actions were natural to which class of people. When the *Bhagavad Gita* declares that death in pursuit of one's own *dharma* is preferable to following someone else's *dharma,* it relies on this *guna* theory as the basis of differences in personal dispositions to action.

In a classic analysis of the caste system in India, the French anthropologist Louis Dumont showed that the hierarchy of status and power is inherent in the dynamics of castes. The desirability of purity and the danger of pollution keep high castes apart from the low.[16] At the heart of the matter, though, is human dignity: the extent of humiliation and subjugation in this system is astounding. If, as theory held, the differences between a brahmin and an untouchable were natural and not socially constructed, their inequality was unalterable. A particular untouchable might be able to transform himself to some degree, but the laws governing marriage, the partaking of food, and the choice of occupations insured that groups of people would remain inferior. From the times of the *dharmashastras,* civil and criminal law applied differently to brahmin and *shudra,* and not until recently (at least on the books) has the criminal justice system treated them equally.

It has been argued that the perspective of equality is not Indian. Indeed it is not. Social reform movements in India have borrowed moral values from the outside. The Sikh religion borrowed from Islam the idea of brotherhood and the abolition of *sati* (widow-burning, discussed below), and more recently the Gandhian movement to eradicate untouchability showed Western influence. To many scholars, the Indian constitution and the changes promoted by secularism presented ideas alien to Indian culture.[17]

Secularism in the West means that in political and economic life, and before the law, individuals of different faiths will not be treated differently. But the Indian problem is that even those who believe in the same God are essentially different and unequal. These inequalities flow from the religious tradition itself.

SACRAMENTS AND PASSAGES

As the community was divided into classes, individual life was seen as a set of stages, each ushered in with rituals of passage, each entailing distinct obligations. *Samskara* (literally, "making anew") may be defined as a sacrament of passage. Every *samskara* is regarded as a transforming action that "refines" and "purifies" the living body, "initiating it into new statuses and relationships by giving it a new birth."[18] The number of *samskaras* varies according to different authorities, eras, regions, and castes. But they extend from conception to death, and each alters the nature of a person.

A man's life (and the focus *was* on men) consisted of four stages. Arbitrarily divided into segments of twenty-five years each, life proceeded from a first stage of apprenticeship or studenthood, characterized by celibacy, learning, and preparation for a life informed by traditional obligations; to a second of householdership, whose principal objectives were to create a family and earn a livelihood; to a third stage of forest-dwelling, a retirement preparing one for detachment from worldly processes; and finally that of renunciation, in which all identity and possessions were given up in austere preparation for physical dissolution and spiritual liberation. In practice, the third and fourth stages of life were ideal stages, rarely entered by the masses. Even the lawgivers attached greatest importance to the householding stage, after which the apprenticeship stage was next in importance. Some people, however, never entered the stage of a householder, as others never left it.

The attention of Hindu lawgivers was focused much more on the duties and obligations of men than on those of women. Although the texts address marriage, sexuality, reproduction, and widowhood, the lives of men are more central. Rules for women often follow from their connection with men, a development that plagues the tradition to the present day. Members of the lowest caste, the *shudras*, were, like women, not regarded as fit to receive the sacraments.

It is unclear how often the prescribed *samskaras* are performed in India today. Processes of modernization (especially in urban India) have overwhelmed them. Today even when performed most are abbreviated. From the time these sacraments were first practiced, there were numerous variations and alternatives. Penances were prescribed for omissions, but alternatives including collapsing and truncating were suggested. Allowance was made for the law of distress, which allowed for dispensations in extenuating circumstances. In modern India one finds a spectrum of compliance from high orthodoxy to near neglect of the *samskaras*, with a small amount of money donated to a brahmin taking their place as a penance. Not surprisingly, the sacraments of birth, initiation (among brahmins), marriage, and death are the most enduring.

BIRTH AND INITIATION

The sacraments begin with the conception of life itself. Foods that are regarded as enhancing conception and symbolizing the body of the child are eaten before the couple proceed to ritual intercourse (the *Brihadaranyaka Upanishad* describes the ritual in detail).[19] The earliest texts show a preference for male progeny, and a special ritual *(pumsavana)* was observed toward that end. Because it took place during pregnancy, we may infer that the ancients had knowledge of embryology, in particular, knowledge of when sexual differentiation in the embryo would be visible.

Simanta (literally "the parting of hair") is a rite retained today among groups and in many regions of India. This ritual symbolizes safe delivery. Performed in the early part of pregnancy, the rite is a social occasion, a public declaration of the pregnancy. A number of other rites deal with the protection of pregnancy.

The next major sacrament is at birth, *jatakarma*. The *Brihadaranyaka Upanishad* enjoins the father to take the newborn son in his lap, offer oblations in the sacred fire, and chant mantras. He was then to breathe into the child's ear the word *speech* and have him lick a mixture of curds, clarified butter, and honey from a golden spoon. After being given a Vedic name, the son was handed to his mother, who then put him to her breast. The rite was usually performed before the umbilical cord was cut.[20] The symbolic giving of the father's "breath" and of special food imparted to the son the spirit and the body of the father and his ancestors (who were also invoked and fed) before he was born free into the world (before the cord was severed), thus connecting the newborn with his lineage. In this sacrament the celebration of a son is explicit, as is the idea of generational continuity through males.

Later texts describe the rite with minor variations in detail, but they are essentially similar. Members of the family pray for a long life and prosperity on behalf of the son, who will enhance family and forefathers through his life. In later practices, preparations are made for the goddess of destiny, who appears on the sixth day to "write the son's future" on his forehead. The exact time of birth (defined as the appearance of the nose from the birth canal) is also to be noted, so that a horoscope can be accurately produced. Sons born at an inauspicious moment according to astrological calculations were regarded as injurious to the life of the father, and in some later injunctions the father was not to see the son for eighteen years (if he was not abandoned earlier).[21] Other sacraments follow the parturition rite: the giving of the name, the first solid feeding, tonsure, and so on.

Before the investiture of the sacred thread, which leads to the study of the Vedas and *dharma,* the rules of purity do not apply to the child. From the time he is breastfed until the time he begins to take solid foods, the infant is not made impure by contact with his menstruating mother. Being only milkfed, the infant preserves his purity. And during this stage contact with his excrement does not pollute the mother.

A prolonged physical intimacy between mother and child assures later sharing, togetherness and an ability to assimilate. Speaking of infants and children in India, child analyst Lois Murphy wrote,

> Their experience is predominantly an experience of being *with* the rest of the family. . . . This constant togetherness and participation may mean that the small child is rarely exposed to new experiences without the support of a trusted person; it also provides an experience of kinesthetic and empathic richness which children brought up in cribs, playpens, carriages and other articles of furniture could not possibly have. The child comes to know and feel and intuitively to understand people with a depth grown from the time he is close to muscles and bodies, the movements and the feelings of people, just as our children learn to understand the mechanics of objects through the hours and days they spend playing with, taking apart and putting together the objects which are their toys and their vehicles."[22]

The early childhood of Indian boys is generally very permissive and what Westerners might regard as indulgent. The young parents, and especially the mother, experience a change in their status with the birth of a son, a prized possession. Breastfeeding goes on long after dentition, and weaning usually occurs abruptly with the birth of the next child. Toilet training is begun early and occurs over a long period to promote the natural growth of sphincter control in an atmosphere of encouragement. During this period a child is regarded as totally innocent, and ordinary rules of conduct do not apply. There is an unconditional regard for the son, with no blame or punishment for infraction of rules. This changes abruptly at the time of initiation. Suddenly conditions of worth are imposed as the son moves from the nurturing and gratifying domain of mother and other female relatives to the world of the father, the teacher, and other men.[23] The only significant male who remains indulgent is the maternal uncle.

The initiation ceremony demarcates a special transition. A similar shift in regard occurs at about the time of entering school, the first venture into the world outside the family. The contrasting attitudes at this critical juncture in the development of a boy signify the chasm between the home and those outside.[24]

With the rite of initiation the men of the upper castes are born again. *Upanayana*—that which leads one into study of the Vedas and toward fulfilling the obligations of *dharma*—re-forms a person through various ceremonial rituals. In the brahminical tradition initiation was a central rite of passage. The removal of impurities thus far acquired and the generation of new qualities appropriate to religious learning became over time a more or less exclusive ritual of the brahmins. Though Vedic study is no longer undertaken nor is the rite performed at the age of entering school, the *upanayana* continues to be a major occasion in the life of a brahmin. The performance of the sacrament before marriage is mandatory.

The *upanayana* has three crucial parts: the receiving of the sacred *gayatri* hymn (symbolic of the learning of the Vedas, as the hymn occurs in the *Rig Veda*), receiving a staff (symbolic of the life of a mendicant, who was enjoined to beg for his food), and the investiture of the sacred thread (symbolic of an upper garment).[25]

The life of a student was austere and usually celibate. He was to focus on learning, serve the teacher, tend the sacred fire, and bring the teacher food. The only explicit reference to sexual restraint was the major sin of defiling the teacher's bed. Opposition to a long apprenticeship (well into adulthood) was based on the Vedas' injunction that men become householders and have children. One text ridiculed overextended studenthood by suggesting that such students were only trying to hide their impotence.[26]

During this phase, the student followed dietary guidelines. Foods regarded as exciting were avoided, and those regarded as calming and cooling were preferred. Aside from studying the Vedas, the student learned a variety of codes of conduct. For instance, he was taught how to greet someone with all the permutations possible, depending on the other person's place in a hierarchy in relation to the student.

In the modern *upanayana* rites I have observed in Gujarat, the reenactment of the young boy's departure to the home of a teacher and his entrance into the life of an acolyte is equated with renunciation of worldly objectives. The acolyte, head shaven, staff in hand, runs away after receiving his sacred thread, and his maternal uncle runs after him. When the boy's hiding place is discovered, the uncle cajoles him with promises of gifts into returning to regular life. One of the ritual temptations is the promise of a beautiful bride.

Departure from the house of his teacher is an occasion of great importance. Mythology as well as current belief and practice puts a premium on repayment for the teacher's services. *Gurudakshina*, giving to the teacher what one owes him, is an emotionally charged obligation. The Hindu epics have celebrated the teacher's right to demand whatever he thinks appropriate. The *Mahabharata* has it that Drona, the arch-teacher in the epic, asked for the right thumb of an archery student (who learned archery by receiving inspiration from a statue of the legendary teacher). He did this to ensure that the student in question would not surpass another student, the teacher's favorite. This is a story that most children in India learn, as I did in my preteen years.

The one who departs from the house of the teacher at graduation is a *snataka*. He has to lead a pure life, not exposing himself to sexual excitement, speaking the truth but also that which is agreeable, not speaking disagreeable truths nor agreeable lies, and not looking at naked women except in intercourse.[27] The *shastras* include a myriad of rules in exhaustive detail: rules for worship and prayer, salutation, apparel, conduct in crossing rivers, and so on. There is no differentiation between the secular and the spiritual, the essential and the nonessential.

MARRIAGE AND FAMILY LIFE

From the Vedas to modern manuals, the life stage of the householder has been celebrated.

Vivaha, taking away in a special manner, or *parinaya*, going around the sacred fire, were wedding ceremonies readying a man for the performance of the ancient domestic sacrifice and for the begetting of sons who would maintain a generational link with the forefathers.[28] It is unclear whether the act of completing oneself as a man was accomplished by acquiring a wife or by acquiring sons through her. In any case she was essential.

Over time, the marriage ceremony has acquired the accretions of local custom, the great tradition interpenetrating with local traditions. Considerations of time, status, class, caste, family, and the needs of the couple have given the wedding rites every possible twist.

Traditionally the marriage is contracted between families, not between bride and groom. The major prohibition is against the two sharing a common lineage.[29] Marriages between two people with sufficiently divergent family origins, such as separate subcastes, are condemned. A prospective bride or groom is closely examined and may be ruled out if diseases like mental illness, epilepsy, or leprosy are part of the family history. After the basic taboos have been excluded and practical qualifications concerning age, beauty, intelligence, and health have been considered, the proper astrological conjunctions must be ascertained.

"Marriage is a symbolic action that creates a new family by uniting the separate and previously unrelated bodies of a man and a woman into a single body." A wife is referred to as half of one's body. Some traditions emphasize the differences between the wife's substance and the husband's. In Bengal, the expression goes that to join the husband's lineage is as difficult for the new wife as cooking iron beans (she is to some extent alien until she bears a son and merges the bloodlines).[30]

Ritual purification, the sacred fire, the joining of hands, the symbolic mixing of bodies and lineages, and the act of walking around the fire are the most common features of a wedding ceremony. The "seven steps" are the marriage vows: first for becoming one, second for vigor, third for prosperity, fourth for pleasure, fifth for progeny, sixth for favorable seasons, and seventh for friendship.

The family is also the *samsara* of a particular person. It is the spread of kin related by blood, sometimes three generations. When the father is alive, his sons often live in the same house with their wives and children. Some maintain a separate kitchen for each son under the same roof, some a separate pot of money. Even those who do not share a household tend to consult each other in important family transactions. Decision making usually means deferral to the elders. The extended family is the norm in India, and sons who have moved away to work and maintain a separate household regard themselves as part of this larger family. The major tasks of the extended family are regulation of competition and achievement of harmony.

An Indian child grows up in a home filled with people. All manner of paternal relatives, even if not a part of the household, are present almost constantly, and maternal relatives also abound. The Indian dwelling is built to accommodate the flow of people and thus lacks the privacy of a Western home. One room opens into another, a passage through the next a necessity. A child's relationship with his or her own parents is not exclusive, but the recognition and relationship are explicit. The family puts a premium on togetherness, and affiliation is the desired norm.[31] Getting along, even at a personal cost, and making solidarity a cause larger than oneself are primary requirements of the system.

The relationship between brothers is formal, governed by rules of respect and deference. The brother-sister relationship, however, is warm, affectionate, and informal. A sister who leaves the parental home to become part of her husband's family maintains a tender tie to her original home. As a mother's and father's day is observed in the United States, the Hindus celebrate a sister's and a brother's day.

Although the new constitution forbids polygamy for Hindus, polygamy was not forbidden by traditional Hindu law. Indeed, a man was *required* to take a second wife if the first was diseased or childless, particularly sonless. But according to dharmic law a man could not abandon his previous wife; there was no provision for divorce. Under no circumstances was a wife allowed to take a second husband. Adultery was also common, and sanctions against it varied according to context.

Given the complexity of Indian society (in terms of the varying degrees to which groups were within the mainstream of Hindu tradition, and the lack of a church, a book, or a priestly order), these legal provisions were observed irregularly. In some tribal, near-tribal, and lower-caste groups the customs and laws regarding marriage and divorce vary a great deal. Brahminical law was applied and accepted by the three upper castes (the *kshatriya* and *vaishya* castes emulated the brahmin elite as a way of upgrading themselves). This logic applied especially to monogamy, avoidance of divorce, observance of rites, and vegetarianism.

AGING

The great tragedy of the epic *Ramayana* begins with the king's discovery of a few gray hairs while looking in the mirror. Then and there he decides that it is time to quit the throne, hand over the reins to his eldest son, and retire to the forest. The *smriti* literature has the same criterion for retirement, the appearance of gray hair. The stage of forest-dwelling was also said to begin when a man's son had sons. The son with his own family was ready to take over the familial and religious obligations, and the father was free to pursue a life of solitude and contemplation.

In the literature we find examples of forest dwellers, but there is more emphasis on *sannyasins*, or renouncers. The *sannyasin* was supposed to be the last stage of life, although some took *sannyasa* vows before passing through the other stages. This effort consisted in relinquishing all forms of social identification, including one's *jati* (subcaste), one's sacred thread, and even one's name. The *sannyasin* could not own property or be recognized by his family or anyone else. He was legally dead. Even at death, having lost his identity, he ws buried rather than cremated like most other Hindus. Because he had no ties to the body, he needed no separation from it by fire.

Giving up attachments and identity were preparation for that final departure. The fate of the departed was a matter of great concern, and lengthy preparation to ensure a favorable outcome was crucial in the last two life stages. For ordinary folk, the loss of vigor and vitality was a major preoccupation. The medical literature as well as some of the sacrificial rites attest to attempts at rejuvenating the flagging body. Loss of sexual appetite and performance was at the heart of anxiety connected with the processes of aging.

One of the main Ayurvedic texts, the *Carakasamhita*, includes two specialties, the chemistry of rejuvenation and the science of increasing virility. As in most other matters, these efforts are directed toward men rather than women. We may surmise that men were more vulnerable and fragile, in greater danger of losing their sexual prowess. Women, on the other hand, have been seen from ancient to modern times as inexhaustible in their sexual appetites. After all, it was men who gave up their vitality (semen) to women.

DEATH AND DYING

From the beginning Hindu civilization has grappled with the problem of death. Interpreting the experience of death was a principal motive of the Upanishadic literature. The idea of a self "free from old age, from death and grief, from hunger and thirst" and the doctrines of rebirth and transmigration are products of that effort.[32] The idea of dying at a ripe old age after long preparation ceased to evoke profound anxiety. For that matter death was preferable to a life of disease and decrepitude. But death does not come only at ripe old age. Untimely death causes fear and sorrow among those left behind.

Hindus do not look on death as only a personal event. The mourning family participates both before (when expected) and after the mortal end of life with great sorrow and grief. The children lose the protection of the father or the elder or the love of the mother, and when a young person (especially a son) dies there is no end to the parents' misery. When a man dies, his widow suffers serious consequences. It is best to die after the debts to gods, sages, and ancestors have been paid. Death is not the opposite of life, it is the opposite of birth, the two events marking passage through the cycle of births.

Hindus are generally cremated, both because fire purifies that which is impure and because fire most effectively returns bodies to their original form. In cremation the body is offered to the fire, and the ashes then are given to the holy waters; performance of this rite is a major obligation of survivors. Children who die before dentition, or before the *upanayana* rite, are considered to be pure; they, along with the renouncers, are accorded burial. In the lower castes burial is also the norm.

KARMA AND REBIRTH

In the course of life, flowing from birth to death and then on to other births and deaths, the theory of *karma* (action) not only connects one life with the next but also provides the ethical grounds for action. That an act has a meaning beyond its apparent and immediate consequence and that actions connect the actor with past and future events serve to explain particular life courses. The origins of the theory of *karma* and rebirth are as old as the Indian civilization. It has been suggested that these theories evolved among the inhabitants of the land before the arrival of the Aryans. Later the ideas were incorporated into Hindu Vedic and post-Vedic thought.[33]

Karma has three dimensions: past, present, and future. What is happening now is a result of deeds in the past, and what was done is unalterable. But in the present one has choices: good and ethical actions result in future events that bring happiness and comfort, alleviation of misery and sorrow. There are actions yet to be undertaken and they, like the acts in the present, provide an opportunity to alter one's fate. Generally interpreted as fatalistic, the *karma* theory actually provides incentives for "good works" and a way of determining the future.

In this scheme the idea of rebirth explains ordinarily inexplicable events. Why do some die young, why are others born with defects, and still others born in a low caste or consigned to poverty and misery? The causes are said to be actions in a past life for which just punishments are borne in this birth. Unusual gifts and talents, unexpected good fortune, wealth and well-being, and virtuous conduct also have their antecedents in a previous life.

Karma and rebirth are answers to the "why me?" questions of people in general and patients in particular. What is unexpected, accidental, or not easily explained in terms of cause and effect is usually attributed to the unseen hand of *karma*. In their everyday thinking, Indians do not generally ponder the karmic significance of their actions; they are neither propelled into nor inhibited from good or bad acts, except in specific religious observances. More commonly when things don't turn out as expected, *karma* is invoked as an explanation. Helplessness produced by disease and death is relieved by belief in the accumulation of past deeds.

We may say that *dharma* (duty) ordains action and *karma* attempts to hold a person to a particular course. Actions derive their moral content from their accord with the *dharma* of a particular person at a particular time. Hindu ethics is governed by a theory of temporality and action that extends beyond one human lifetime. The most important accounting of action occurs at the end of a lifetime, for the casting into the next birth is determined by the balance on the ledger of *karma*.

At death what survives are the *atman,* the undecaying, disembodied consciousness, and the *jiva,* the life principle. Together as the *jivatman* they are freed from the body. The *jiva* is the repository of the record (residues) of actions that determines the course of *jivatman* after a death.

The supreme goal after the release from the body is to be freed from *samsara* altogether, to attain *moksha* or liberation from rebirth. The fate of the *atman* in this eventuality would be a merger with the ultimate reality *(brahman)* from which it once arose. But the road to liberation is difficult, its destination not to be hoped for by ordinary people. It requires of a person acts of extreme austerity that close all avenues of input and output, causing thirst and hunger to waste the body away. Ordinary men and women have to settle for second best and take precautions against intermediate fates or lowly rebirths. Knowing the path to *moksha* but not being able to pursue it is attributed to the power of attachments *(maya).*

In Hindu eschatology there are three fates intermediate between life and the bliss of *moksha.* "All who depart from this world (or this body) go to the moon."[34] The moon is a way station, a place for processing, from which some go on to the land of forefathers (Pitriloka). Here the dead wait for a body to be supplied by their sons, who discharge their filial duty in the *shraddha* ceremony, discussed below. When newly embodied they are released from their temporary abode and return to earth. A third and undesirable fate for the departed is not to reach the land of the fathers but to roam the earth in search of fulfillment. The *pretas* are disembodied *jivatmas* who have failed to ascend to Pitriloka and become ghosts, either because their sons failed to give them a body to live in or because their earthly desires were so strong, their passions so unsated, and their ambitions so unrealized that they must enter another person's body to fulfill them. Roaming unsated *pretas* can take over, or possess, human bodies in states of impurity or vulnerability.

The *shraddha* rite is considered by almost all Hindus the most important obligation of a son to his father and forefathers, perhaps even the most important obligation in life.[35] (There are conflicting edicts regarding the *shraddha* ceremony to be performed for the mother and her ancestors, but in some families, including mine, the ceremonies are performed for paternal relations of the mother and for the mother as well.) The ceremony consists of preparing ten balls of cooked rice mixed with milk. The balls of rice are called *pinda,* meaning an embryo but generally referring to the whole bodily frame. (There are corrupt versions of the word in modern Indian languages that mean the body.) The son is often called "the roller of rice balls." The verses recited during the ten-day process explicitly constitute the body of the dead father which was cremated; the number ten represents the ten lunar months of pregnancy. The body so made is then cooled with water, oil, and a certain grass. Flowers and colored powders contribute smell and form, the sacred thread is added as clothing, and then the son completes the dead father by blowing his "breath" into the body. Later in the ceremony three large balls of rice (representing the three previous generations) are rolled, and one large ball (for all of the ancestors) is mixed with the body of the father.[36] The rite presumes a oneness between the father and the son: the son gives a body to the father as the father had once given him a body. A modern translation may be, "I am because you were, and you will be because I am." In turn the reconstituted father produces progeny for the son, as the eating of the balls of rice by the wife of the son will produce a son for her.

Hindu *samsara*, the flowing life, is bounded by the sacraments presaging transitions and passages, and time is stretched to infinity by a law of action and its consequences. Hindu laws attempt to provide coherence and continuity, thus giving shape to life that is prone to change and ultimately fragile. Over the centuries of the Indian past, the struggle with the unanswerable questions of life and death and the consequent anxiety have been dealt with by a series of accommodations. The idea of an interior and undying self and a natural law of action have bound persons internally as well as in external social transactions. On one hand life is fluid, but the individual is also aware of well-defined channels and vessels. At times the channels and vessels have become rigid, unable to accommodate the tides of change; therein may lie the orthodoxy and persistence of patterns of Hindu life and ethos.

· 4 ·

The Self

When the sun has set and the moon has set, and the fire is gone out, and the sound hushed, what is then the light of man?
The Self indeed is his light.

Brihadaranyaka Upanishad

Constructs of the self and the body are at the heart of a tradition's intersection with its medical enterprise. Experiences of pain and suffering come through the body and are translated through the awareness of being a person. A culture is shaped by the assumptions of its faith traditions, as the traditions are organized by the historical antecedents of that culture. These dynamics repose in the notion of what it is to be a person, in an inner sense of continuity and coherence. Nowhere is the need to examine the beliefs about "I-ness" more important than in the Indian traditions, for the culture has been preoccupied with a search for the definition and meaning of selfhood from its beginnings. In their intellectual and philosophical pursuits, the Hindus have fashioned an understanding of the self as the "I" encased in a body, which stands in marked contrast to Western constructions—religious, medical, and psychological.

Realization of authentic selfhood may be regarded as the cornerstone of Hindu experience. Hindu religious thought turns to the idea of a self for both a ground of meaning and a sense of continuity in all eventualities (birth and death, pain, suffering, and old age) and all life-tasks (work, procreation, relationships, learning, healing, and worship).

From its beginnings, Hindu speculations about the nature of the self have been grounded in materiality. Even when in the later development of Hindu thought the ideas turn to more abstract constructions, the self remains tethered to its original ground. Duality between a material self and a transcendental self (akin to some Western definitions of the soul) does emerge, but the opposition between the two is a matter more of distinction than of antagonism. Unlike the division between Greek psyche and soma,

35

Hindu mind and body are material and confluent. The self on the other hand is partitioned into a transcendental or spiritual self, *atman*, and the phenomenal self, *ahamkara*. *Atman* is more private, *ahamkara* more public. In the spiritual and ethical realms, *atman* is more positively valenced, nearer to and more like God, *ahamkara* more negatively valenced, more worldly and human.

These ideas are central to an understanding of Hindu self-experience, especially in fathoming the experience of death and dying. Though the early Hindu poets and philosophers celebrated the experience of being alive and exulted in their discovery of selfhood, they were gripped with melancholy in the face of death, an inevitability that finally shaped their ideas about an undecaying self.

This chapter examines these concepts of the self and their origins and development. Early Hindu literature, the Vedas and Upanishads, are the major sources of the study. Later developments, specifically those relevant to the foundations of health and medicine, will also be presented.

CREATION, FRAGMENTATION, AND REINTEGRATION

Hindu literature presents several slightly different renderings of the creation of life, in keeping with the Hindu spirit of not granting absolute power or absolute meaning to anything. As the Vedic hymns make clear, the first creative impulse was to unite humankind with the forces of nature and gods. Later speculation led to myths of the origin of the human race and the cosmos. The "Nasadiya" hymn is indeed speculative, filled with uncertainty, casting doubt on the creator himself, but principally adhering to the theme of ineffability in the act of creation. Here we come upon desire as the first seed:

> Neither not-being nor being was there at that time: there was no air-filled space nor was the sky which is beyond it. What enveloped all? And where? Under whose protection? What was the unfathomable deep water? . . .

> Neither was death there, nor even immortality at that time; there was no distinguishing mark of day and night. That one breathed without wind in its own special manner. Other than it, indeed, and beyond, there did not exist anything whatsoever. . . .

> In the beginning there was darkness concealed in darkness; all this was an indistinguishable flood of water. That which, possessing life-force, was enclosed by Vacuum, the One, was born through the power of heat from its austerity. . . .

Upon It, rose up, *in the beginning, desire, which was the mind's first seed.*
Having sought in their hearts, the wise ones discovered through delibera-
tion, the bond of being and non-being. . . .

Wherefrom this creation has issued, whether he has made it or whether he
has not—he who is the superintendent of this world in the highest
heaven—he alone knows, or, perhaps, even he does not know.[1]

For the Rig Vedic poets, creation is an act of desire equivalent to self-
consciousness, a consciousness that separates the unity of man with nature, a
falling apart. To repair and heal this disjunction, the Rig Vedic ritual identifies a single giant, the cosmic man Purusha, as the performer of a sacrificial
ritual that accomplishes unity with the Creator. Birth and death are interpreted as the opening and closing of the world, attributed to the acts of this
ordainer of the cosmic order. Purusha, a differentiated entity, arises from an
undifferentiated, uncertain, and undefinable matrix, *brahman*.[2]

There are a variety of creation mythologies in Hindu literature, which
become less uncertain and less abstract as divine and human become more
separate.

In another creation hymn a golden embryo is thought to have preceded
all.[3] The speculative "who," the creator, is given a name. The context is
human, and the images of seed, egg, and womb are transparent, tied to the
birth of a god who at the beginning is nameless and thus undifferentiated but
clearly linked to creation and procreation. In the last verse of this hymn, we
suddenly have a name: Prajapati. The name is connected to generativity—
the lord *(pati)* of beings *(praja)*.

Next we turn to the "Purushasukta" hymn, occurring in the late *Rig Veda*.[4]
In this hymn, the body of Purusha is broken down into parts which become
the elements: his breath becomes the wind, his eyes the sun. In other texts
he becomes the foundation of social order, the castes: his mouth becomes the
priest; his arms become the warriors; his thighs become the commoner; and
from his feet is born the toiler. The dismemberment of this giant into the
parts that constitute the universe invests the hymn with the immensity of
both the power of creation and the tragedy of disintegration.

Mythologist Joseph Campbell, in comparing this creation myth with the
biblical version, observes that in the Genesis story

> God and Man, from the beginning, are distinct. Man is made in the image
> of God, indeed, and the breath of God has been breathed into his nostrils;
> yet his being, his self, is not that of God, nor is it one with the universe.
> The fashioning of the world, of the animals, and of Adam (who then became
> Adam and Eve) was not accomplished within the sphere of divinity but

outside of it. There is consequently an intrinsic, not merely a *formal*, separation.

"Moreover," Campbell continues, "it was only after creation that man fell; whereas in the Indian example, creation itself was a fall—the fragmentation of God."[5]

In the Vedic myth, the god poured himself forth into beings, because of his desire to propagate and extend himself. In the Hebrew version, too, it was desire that led to the fall; but it was the desire of the created humans, not that of the creating god. In the biblical version as interpreted by the apostle Paul, humans must repent to be saved. In the Hindu account, the falling apart is both creative and tragic; humans yearn for reunification, the reconstitution of the original whole, the *brahman*, of which they are themselves a part *(atman)*.

Concerns about creativity, procreativity, and dissolution are prominent in Indian consciousness today. If the life of the primordial person Prajapati (the most common appellation of Purusha) is taken as paradigmatic for humans, we can distill several Hindu assumptions about the human situation. In the cosmogony of the Vedic Hindus and in the sacrificial ritual that was designed to recreate the primordial events (thereby uniting the performers of the sacrifice with cosmic forces), there is an explicit attempt to gain control over the perpetual alternation in the workings of the universe.[6] When the sacrificial rituals failed to allay the anxieties of the Vedic Hindus, they tried to internalize the cosmic man so that the union between humankind and the cosmos would be complete. The internalized version was also called the *atman*, as when the poets pronounced: "This *atman* is *brahman*." In the later Vedic literature the cosmic principle was placed within the person; a thumb-sized version of the cosmic person resided within the heart.

The Vedic texts celebrate the prolific creativity of Prajapati, and all living and nonliving substances emanated from his dismemberment. For example, the five parts into which Prajapati disintegrated were hair, skin, flesh, bone, and marrow. In other texts he also fell apart into five seasons and five regions of space. In the spirit of a sacrificial ritual, which is the main subject of the *brahmanas*, the sacrificer is told to heat the offerings on a golden plate and add kindling sticks in order to put breath, vigor, and food back into himself. The strategy is to allay the fears of dissolution. The texts also dwell on the relationship between Prajapati and his son Agni. They enhance each other, but more particularly the son restores the father's integrity and cohesion.

In summary, the Rig Vedic texts address the problems of creation, fragmentation, and reintegration. The Vedic gods preside over different realms of the universe and have to be appeased so that they will grant boons rather than bring destruction. The cosmos is experienced as governed by law, by the *rita* which is awe-inspiring and at the same time beneficent in forming an order on which the human heart rests. The body itself is a repository for these divine powers. A primordial person is conceived by waters and in turn emits all of creation through falling apart. The substances of which the cosmos and humanity are composed are the very substances of which the primordial person was made, and reintegration of the weakly structured person becomes a central concern of the later texts. Death, and thus disintegration, is overshadowed by the celebration of prolific creativity.

THE UPANISHADS: SELF AS BREATH

As the metaphysicians described the meaning and essence of life, they went from the immediate experience of life, rooted in their self-perceptions and observations, to an abstract, theoretical, and psychologically informed construct of the essence of life, the *atman*.

Generally regarded as commentaries on the Vedas, the Upanishads, which number close to 150, span a long period: mainly several centuries before and after the Buddha's lifetime (ca. 563–483 B.C.E.).[7] The Upanishadic authors were in search of truths they could transmit to successive generations, often presenting their arguments in the form of dialogues between teachers and pupils or fathers and sons. The line of arguments they used left little doubt either about their quest to understand the essence and meaning of life or about their method, which was rooted in observation and introspection. In their observations about life, they drew much from trying to understand death (and in their introspection discovered a sense of selfhood as the essential "I-ness").[8] Their turn toward what has been regarded as the mystical can only be so designated if one neglects the path they took in reaching their goal.

In early Hindu thought the concept of self was associated with the breath. When writers spoke of *prana*, they spoke of breath alone in the material sense and then distinguished types of breath such as inhalation and exhalation. They later widened the definition of *prana* to encompass "wind" in different parts of the body, which crystallized into the idea of a vital force or *jiva* (often translated as soul).

Prana (breath) is the essential characteristic of life, and thus the departure of *prana* is synonymous with death, as in the colloquial expression "the *prana* has flown away."[9] Many other expressions in the English language, like "waiting with bated breath" or "holding one's breath," find parallels in

Hindu expressions—"I was afraid my breath left me" or "my breath disappeared into my palate" (usually meaning the inside of the head). In the *Brihadaranyaka Upanishad* the various senses and body functions vie with each other for first place. The breath, the eyes, the ears, the mind, the seed—each in its own right has a significant function, but claims to priority and dominance are not easily settled. In one story, they go to Brahman to have their argument settled. "Who is the richest of us?" they ask. Brahman (or Prajapati in the *Chandogya Upanishad*) replies: "He by whose departure this body seems worst, he is the richest." Each of the senses in turn leaves the body. Speech leaves a person without the ability to speak, but the rest of the functions go on. Similarly, loss of eyes results in blindness, ears in deafness, mind in foolishness, and seed in loss of generative capacity. Finally, it comes to breath, which "on the point of departure, tore up these senses, as a great, excellent horse of the Sindhu country might tear up the pegs to which he is tethered. They said to him: 'Sir, do not depart. We shall not be able to live without thee.'"[10]

Often the word *prana* is used generically for the sense organs; the authors then distinguish between ordinary *pranas*, or the senses, and the vital *prana*, the breath. *Vayu*, the cosmic element of which the breath is an extension, is regarded as the agent of the union between heaven and earth.[11] Food, which so preoccupied these early settlers on the Indian subcontinent, competes often with breath for preeminence. Food is a condition for life, from which all creatures are produced, from which they derive nourishment, without which growth is not possible and also to which all beings return. But the "inner self, which consists of breath," is different from food and "consists of the essence of food."[12] The poets praise breath as the "essence of the body parts." That *prana* is not an immaterial entity is made explicit by references to it as the "lord of speech" and as "that which comes from the mouth."

Several stories establish the centrality of breath. In the *Brihadaranyaka Upanishad*, the body parts are threatened by deities explicitly equated with evil and called Death. The body parts are saved by *prana*, however, and then taken to their origin.[13] Breath, which "eats" food, is seen to nourish the various body parts. The Upanishadic poets explain the "withering" of the limb (wasting occasioned perhaps by paralysis) as the "going-away of the breath" from that limb.[14] Thus breath is also called *angirasa*, the sap of the limbs.[15]

The authors of the Upanishads later introduce another dimension of breath. Breath now unites and connects the body parts of a person. "Prajapati created the actions (active senses). When they had been created, they strove among themselves. The voice held, I shall speak; the eye held, I shall see; the ear held, I shall hear; and thus other actions too, each according to its own act. Death, having become weariness, took them and seized them. Having seized them, Death held them back (from their work). Therefore, speech grows weary, the eyes grow weary, the ears grow weary."[16] But breath was not seized because it could not be seized. The other faculties took refuge in breath and assumed its form, thus defying death. *Prana* here is that which makes the parts into a cohesive whole. The connecting function of breath is illustrated in yet another metaphor, a thread that strings together. A dead person's limbs come unstrung.[17]

Hindus from early on have distrusted all that was not stable. Life itself is one such thing. The principle of *rita*, the rule that governs the universe in an orderly fashion, becomes an early abstraction that generates veneration. The moon waxes and wanes, the sun sets. The moon and the sun obey the *rita* but do not have the qualities of unblinking permanence. "As it was with the central breath among the breaths, so it was with the Vayu, the wind among the deities. The other deities fade, not Vayu. Vayu is the deity that never sets."[18] In these verses celebrating the preeminence of Vayu—breath—there is also an explanation for the failure of the others. They sang for themselves, for their own pleasure, they were intent on doing their own thing, were self-centered ("the moon held, I shall shine") and preoccupied with their own glory. Not so the wind; he worked invisibly, without grandiosity, for the welfare of others, to unite them into a cohesive whole. The body parts, like the deities from which they arose, were not united because of their narcissistic preoccupation. The principle that united them was outside themselves. Here a consciousness is attributed to body parts, derived from their respective origins and tendency to be autonomous. The Upanishads of themselves make the comparison between the breath as unifier, whose forms other agencies of action (such as eyes, ears, and nose) take and by whose name they will be known, and the head of family who unifies and holds together his clan; it is by his name the family will be known.

Later, after many explorations of the possible meanings, connections, origins, and priority of breath, that concept began to lose some ground. References to a "cavity within," generally interpreted as the heart, become more frequent. We find descriptions of a cavity from which arise many channels carrying vital substances. A thumb-sized human shape is said to reside within this cavity. A cavity inside the skull is also described, likened to an inverted vessel with its mouth pointing downward.[19] These anatomical concerns point to a disquiet that must have plagued the early philosophers in their attempts at locating the seat of the self. For the central question that the Upanishads ask concerns the essential ingredients of life, what distinguishes life and death. And this question must also include self-awareness.

One approach was to recognize *brahman* in everything, especially as the essence of everything. All that one saw and experienced was the abode of the supreme being—including the essence of oneself.[20] In this approach the essential difference between all that is created is obliterated, recalling the early idea of creation as the falling apart of Prajapati.

The *Chandogya Upanishad* tells the story of Svetaketu, who had studied the Vedas for twelve years under an appropriate teacher but still had not grasped the all-pervasive yet special nature of the true and essential. His father uses many analogies to tell him of the multiple forms that true substance takes, yet leaving intact the same essence (honey collected by bees from many different flowers, rivers flowing into the sea and losing their distinctions). Finally he asks his son to break open a fruit of the *nyagrodha* tree and then to break one of the tiny seeds inside.

> "What do you see there?"
> "Not anything, sir."
> The father said: "My son, that subtle substance which you do not perceive there, of that very essence the great *nyagrodha* tree exists. Believe it, my son. That which is the subtle essence, in it all that exists has its self. It is the True. It is the self, and thou, o Svetaketu, art it."[21]

In the famous words "thou art it" (*tat tvam asi*, sometimes translated "that thou art") the philosophers of the *Chandogya Upanishad* sum up the universal and all-permeating nature of the true and its identity with the self of a person.

SELF AS CONSCIOUSNESS (ATMAN)

The questions "Who am I, and where am I going?" arise from self-awareness. The Upanishads sought an answer by exploring sleep and dreams. After all, in sleep one continues to breathe, but one is not aware and does not speak. The *Chandogya Upanishad* says, "When a man sleeps speech goes into breath, so do sight, hearing and mind. Breath indeed consumes them all."[22] But with sleep, self-awareness is also gone. Further speculation on this state of consciousness led the philosophers to classify states of consciousness. When a person sleeps, his or her self (the self of self-awareness) disappears within. A closer connection between breath and self is drawn, and slowly breath begins to lose its original meaning, acquiring the more abstract character of self-awareness. The living self is compared to a bird tied to a string, who tries to fly in every direction but in the end must return to where it is tied. The mind, or the conscious self, has to return to *prana*, for it is attached to the breath as if with a string.[23] In classical Hindu fashion, however, ordinary consciousness is not given priority because it fluctuates. The poet imagines that in deep sleep, when the mind has gone to rest within the breath, the "true" is realized.[24]

The Upanishads are a treasury of great dialogues. One such dialogue is between a king, Janaka Vaideha, and Yagnavalkya, a brahmin sage. The discussion ultimately turns to the nature of the self. The king asks the sage, "When the sun has set and the moon has set, and the fire is gone out, and the sound hushed, what is then the light of man?" We may assume this condition to be sleep or death. In reply, the sage constructs images without sensations and objectless ideas, as in sleeping and dreaming. The self wanders in sleep and creates ponds, lakes, and rivers. In a belief that has survived to the present, we find an Upanishad advising: "Let no one wake a man suddenly, for it is not easy to remedy if he does not get back (rightly to his body)."[25]

The states of consciousness are classified in the *Mandukya Upanishad.* The waking state is explained as a state in which the gross objects of sense are apprehended. In dreaming, the objects are internal, and the movement is from the gross to the subtle. The self is freed from the objects of sensations. Next comes the state of deep sleep or dreamless sleep. This state enjoys a higher place in the hierarchy, for in it there are no objects to be apprehended, external or internal. At this point in the development of Upanishadic thought, *prana* has become significantly detached from its literal meaning. Now pure awareness (awareness only of awareness) dominates the search for answers. Awareness occasioned by sense-perceptions is secondary. A fourth state of consciousness is then hypothesized, *turiya.* In this state consciousness itself is annihilated.[26] The principle of negation, "not this, nor that," an idiom of the Upanishads, is replayed to prove the nature of the self. Many of the yogic practices are an attempt, stage by stage, to create such a state and fathom the nature of consciousness itself.

The *Katha Upanishad* tells a story of a young man, Naciketas, who is given away by his father to the god of death, Yama. The sacrifice is made by the father either out of anger at the son's persistent interruptions, or as a kind of trade with Yama, the son for the father. Naciketas confronts his father, asking to whom he was to be given. The father replies angrily, "To death." The young man then goes to the abode of Yama, who is away, and he spends three nights there without food.

Obliged to treat Naciketas specially to undo the misfortune that would befall a man in whose house a guest stayed without food, Yama therefore grants him three boons. For the first boon Naciketas asks that "my father be pacified, kind, and free from anger towards me; and that he may know me, and greet me, when I shall have been dismissed by thee."[27] This boon permits Naciketas to return from the abode of death, from whence none return, but we glean that a repair in his relationship with his father is uppermost in his mind. In a sense, Yama, the god of death, becomes Naciketas's father, giving him a new birth. Like many heroes of Hindu tales, Naciketas turns to a man other than his father for special knowledge, using his second boon to ask the secret of ascending to heaven. Naciketas wants to know how the fire sacrifice, "the beginning of all the worlds," is performed. Yama not only grants the wish but also names the sacrifice after him. The performers of this sacrifice, Yama says, will henceforth overcome birth and death and rejoice in heaven (attain immortality).

For his third boon Naciketas asks Yama to explain to him the mystery of death. All attempts to dissuade the young man from his request are in vain. The promise of untold wealth or a long life does not deter Naciketas from his desire to unravel the mystery of death. Yama is pleased that the young man has distinguished what is good from what is pleasurable. The rest of the Upanishad dwells on the meaning of the self. The self, ancient, unseen, and subtle, is neither this nor that. It is not a cause, not an effect. Recognized by the syllable *Om*, the highest self is neither born nor dies. It springs from nothing, and nothing springs from it. The heart of the description is that this self, the *atman*, is regarded as that which is not killed when the body is killed.[28]

SELF AS "I-NESS" (*AHAMKARA*)

In the beginning this was self alone, in the shape of a person *(purusha)*. He looking around saw nothing but his Self. He first said, "This is I;" therefore he became "I" by name.[29]

So began the experience and the idea of *ahamkara*. Literally, the utterance of the word *I* (*ahamkara*) came to be designated a kind of self-awareness, the consciousness of being a person. In this cosmogenic passage, the utterance of the word *I* is a cry and triumph of creation. In the gradual unfolding of the self-experience, *ahamkara* was a self-formulation, the realization of selfhood. In their search for the meaning of life which had become equated with the breathing trunk, the authors of the Upanishads became explicit about the nascent self-feeling. The articulation and realization of being a person was a continuous process throughout the early Vedic era, and in *ahamkara* reached a stage in which the definitions of the self required a definition of the other as well.

We may recall that the prolific creativity of Prajapati sprang from desire, the first seed, a wish to propagate himself. This was the first act of self-consciousness—for the wish to propagate oneself, a rich source of transformations, is also an act of narcissistic enhancement. Seeking continuity through one's progeny was a process of fragmentation, giving up a part of oneself to create another, and in the case of Prajapati, a falling apart of the body into parts. Creativity of this sort was intricately linked with tragedy. The experience of *ahamkara* from the very beginning has carried this bivalent meaning.

The *Brihadaranyaka Upanishad* proceeds from the definition above to a further definition of the self. Because the person who was first cannot allow anyone or anything else before him, he burns all that vies for first place. Clearly in this conception the narcissistic aspect of the self is paramount. But then the first person experiences loneliness. He is afraid that another may exist, and hence "fear arises from another. But he had no delight. Therefore a man who is lonely has no delight." We may rephrase this insight as "alone one cannot play, from the second fear comes." The authors of the Upanishads find a unique solution to this dilemma. The original person divides himself into two, a man and a woman, husband and wife, and therefore "We two are thus (each of us) like half a shell."[30] Now the other is a part of oneself and need not be feared. The other is there to give delight, response, self-affirmation.[31]

Thus *ahamkara* is born out of self-consciousness, and with it arises a need for a second. Desire to be the first, desire to propagate, the fear of being alone, and the need for delight in another's eyes are essential components of selfhood. All these qualities become associated with a self that is active, wishing, and wanting. It is full of pride, as in *gaurva*, "swollen and heavy with a sense of self-importance," or as in *smaya*, meaning "the smile of pride of one who receives a compliment or views himself in a mirror."[32]

Attachments are a natural consequence of a wishing and wanting self, but they inevitably produce grief. The need for admiration and affirmation is never quite completely gratified in the world of other *ahamkaras*, responding inadequately from self-interest. A person learns to cope with an unpredictable response to the need for self-enhancement, which leaves the ego-self vulnerable by creating an inner and an outer persona. The behavior of the self operating at two levels of consciousness does not necessarily correspond to inner states. A split-level awareness arises in which the inner self corresponds experientially to the notion of *atman* and an outer self is equated with *ahamkara*.

The nature and meaning of the self, I have argued, was a result of the progressive interiorization of the powers of the cosmos running parallel to, and interacting with, a ceaseless process of introspection into the experience of the self. From its earliest meaning as a purely physical condition of life, breath came to mean a vital force, uniting the body and giving coherence to the self. An earlier meaning of this self as the trunk where breath resides, uniting the other body parts into a whole, is explicit.[33] The Indian folklore of a warrior who continues to fight the enemy even after having been beheaded testifies to the ancient centrality of the trunk. Such a construction renders breath a vital function but does not allow for an understanding of self-awareness. The self then comes to be equated with consciousness, a narcissistic self-awareness. Hindu thought first visualized creation as an act of self-consciousness, the utterance of the word *I*, and later, as a result of the desire to propagate oneself.

The self was next seen as a witness, a sort of pure awareness ultimately freed from all worldly connection except in the role of an observer. This self was untouched by death; the reality of death was defied and denied.

Thus freed, the Self (now uppercase) became the true reality. And so began a dichotomy between the true and false, the latter equated with the worldly and narcissistic component of the self. The freedom so obtained by the true self became a burden for the false one: observer and actor were split apart. The true and prized self was conceived as a part of the divine, while the false self was left behind to carry the body and its psychophysiology.

·5·

The Body

I was once a part of the flow, never thinking of myself a presence. Then I looked in the mirror and decided to be free. All that my freedom has brought me is the knowledge that I have a face and a body, that I must feed this body and clothe this body for a certain number of years. Then it will be over.

V. S. Naipaul, *In a Free State*

For Ayurveda, the Hindu science of life and health, the human body is the primary object of concern. Preservation of life and prevention and alleviation of disease have been explicitly discussed from the earliest times. Body, *sharira,* is that which decays. The anxiety of falling apart is countered with care and attention, and the search for cohesion is central to Hindu medicine.

Body parts and their origins are described in the Vedic literature. Relying on these accounts, the Ayurvedic physicians speculated on body substances (the *dosha*s and *dhatu*s) and their physiology and pathology. How these substances are put together into a whole lies at the center of the relation between tradition and medicine.

THE AYURVEDIC HUMORS

Vata, pitta, and *kapha* are the Ayurvedic humors, the *tridoshas,* and may be translated as wind, bile, and phlegm. Representing movement, heat, and moisture, the three bodily humors govern wellness and illness. The three must be in equilibrium with each other, must be in their appropriate locations, and must be optimally functional. In Ayurvedic pathophysiology diseases of varied etiology are understood through the dynamics of the *tridoshas.*

Ayurvedic texts, otherwise careful and thorough in elucidating the origin of all bodily substances, are curiously silent on how these three humors originated. Such an omission on their part would be puzzling, unless the

47

origin of the humors was obvious. An answer suggests itself if we consider the mainstream of Hindu thought of the Vedic period.

In Vedic times, the gods commanded all spheres of the cosmos and all aspects of human life. All realms, terrestrial and ethereal, natural, social, and personal, were presided over by a particular god who was regarded as the ordainer and regulator of that aspect. No god's power was absolute; all needed to be worshipped to be appeased. Praise was important and extravagant, and nothing was left out of the purview of the gods.

In the Rig Vedic pantheon, Indra is the king and a Zeus-like warrior-god. Hymns proclaim him to be all-powerful, protecting the tribes from all attacks, increasing the herds of their cows, and vanquishing his enemies with his weapon, the thunderbolt; he is identified with thunder, and he controls the rains. The hymns tell of his fight with the demon Vritra. In this myth and its later elaborations Vritra had enclosed the heavens, thus enveloping the waters and the sun. Indra felled the demon and opened the heavens to let the rain fall and dispel the darkness. The closing and the opening of the heavens, a repeated cycle of bondage and release of life-giving substances, became the theme of these very early hymns and the sacrifices that accompanied them. Human beings, who lived in the cosmos that alternated between day and night, between the arid and moist in the summer and monsoon, yearned for the gods' blessings and praised Indra.[1]

The second among the Vedic gods, and equally important, is Agni, the god of fire. In the sacrificial tradition, fire is the center of the ritual. One scholar suggests that Agni has three forms: terrestrial (as fire), atmospheric (as lightning), and celestial (as the sun).[2] Oblations are offered into the sacred fire, and Agni is invoked as the head priest, the one who will carry these offerings to the gods in the heavens. A householder is enjoined always to keep a fire in his home.

Another of the preeminent Vedic gods is Varuna or Vata, the wind god.[3] He moves things, both the celestial and the terrestrial. He also is an ordainer of the natural order, keeping earth and sky apart, and is the guardian of morality.

These gods, however, disappeared from the Hindu pantheon over time. Some scholars have speculated that the qualities these gods represented were absorbed by later Hindu gods who supplanted them,[4] but their disappearance may be more comprehensible in the context of Ayurveda. It seems to me likely that the Vedic gods Varuna, Agni, and Indra were interiorized into the human body, becoming the *vata*, *pitta*, and *kapha* of the Ayurvedic humors. In the humor *vata*, or wind, Varuna took yet another form. Unifying body parts, the wind had the principal characteristic of motion; it moved bodily substances along the designated channels. The fire-god Agni, associated with sacrificial rituals and the hearth, is parallel to *pitta* in the body. *Pitta* (heat) performed the all-important function of cooking the ingested food and thus transformed the food into various constituents usable by the body. *Kapha* (moisture), the third Ayurvedic principle, is derivative of Indra, the king of the earth who opened the heaven to let rain fall.

The three major Vedic gods thus penetrated into the body and the self. What was outside came to reside inside. These gods were partially assimilated and no longer needed to be worshipped. They held sway over the human world, nevertheless, for not all their powers were assimilated. Like the gods who were adored, dreaded, praised, and appeased, the humors were as capable of wreaking havoc as they were of prolonging lines of vigorous progeny, bestowing long life, and augmenting herds of cows. The *dosha*s were responsible for both health and disease. (*Dosha* is often translated as "humor" after the Greek medical tradition, but it means more than just a fluid. From the root *dush*, meaning "a fault, blame, or defect," it carries with it a meaning similar to "sin.") Like the gods from whom they were derived, the humors are capable of benevolence but also malevolence.

CONCEPTS OF THE BODY IN THE UPANISHADS

In the works of the Upanishadic poets and philosophers, the human body became a subject of explicit reflection. Mainly concerned with the principle of life and self-awareness, the authors searched through the functions of the body to arrive at what was essential. In so doing they constructed a physiology of the body, concerning all that was taken in, the possible transformation of all such substances, and their eventual fate (the conversion into essential body constituents and the waste products).

"The essence of all beings is the earth," declares the *Chandogya Upanishad*.[5] It continues by asserting that the essence of the earth is water; the essence of water, plants; and the essence of plants, man; thus establishing a connection between the human body and the earth through water and food. An almost identical passage appears in the *Brihadaranyaka Upanishad*. "The earth is the essence of these things; water is the essence of earth; plants, of water; flowers, of plants; fruits, of flowers; man, of fruits; seed, of man."[6] We understand through these verses the interconnectedness of all things.

The three basic elements have now become five, the *pancha mahabhutas*. Besides wind, fire, and water, they are earth and *akasha*, ordinarily translated as ether. To the Upanishadic scholars, *akasha* represented something far less substantial. "What is the origin of the world? 'Ether'," he replied. "For all beings take their rise from ether and return into ether. Ether is older than these; ether is the rest." In a footnote to this passage, translator F. Max Muller explains, "Ether, or we might translate it, as space, both being intended, however, as names or symbols of the highest Brahman."[7]

The meaning of *akasha* in the Upanishadic literature is not univocal. At times it is equated with breath, but often it is not mentioned at all in the enumeration of the essential qualities. We have to conclude that the experience of *akasha* provoked a sense of mystery, was nebulous, and could not be grasped. Thus it was understood as less material. For example, the *Brihadaranyaka Upanishad* declares that everything except the breath and *akasha* within the body is material, mortal, solid, and finite.[8] This Upanishad offers yet another perspective and equates *akasha* with the heart, as does the *Taittiriya Upanishad*.[9] "Ether (or space) is better than fire. For in the ether exist both sun and moon, the lightning, stars and fire (Agni), through the ether we call, through the ether, we hear, through ether we answer"; thus *Chandogya Upanishad* defines space as that which carries the word.[10] But usually in the Vedic literature, space is seen as infinite and all-pervading. It is subtle and formless and shares many qualities with the wind. The Rig Vedic priests spoke in adoration of the elements and worshipped them as their guardians. In the Upanishads, the forces attained a more material and less ethereal status.

Analogies between the cosmic elements and body parts (especially the senses) are established in the Upanishads. At the very beginning of the *Brihadaranyaka Upanishad*, an analogy is drawn between the cosmos and the body of the sacrificial horse. The horse sacrifice, undertaken to establish the territory of a king, is one of the richest rituals in all of Vedic literature. (Wherever the horse wanders, the local chieftain either surrenders or fights the performer of the sacrifice; eventually, after conquering land in all directions, the horse is sacrificed.) The ritual is also supposed to represent an attempt at rejuvenating a king's failing virility.[11] "Heaven is the back; the sky, the belly; the earth, the chest; the quarters, the two sides; the intermediate quarters, the ribs; the members, the seasons; the joints, months and half-months; the feet, days and nights; the bones, the stars; the flesh, the clouds."

The human counterpart of the body of the sacrificial horse is that of the king. Like the body parts of the horse, the king's are also regarded as equivalent to various aspects of the cosmos. The Upanishads (and such texts as the *Satapatha Brahmana*) repeatedly compare parts of the body to various cosmic elements and regard them as equivalent to these elements and arising out of them. Thus the body parts, though connected, retain the distinctness imparted to them by their origins. The classic equivalence is between the sun and the eye, for example, "the Sun, the eye of the whole world."[12] Eyes shine and have lustre, and like the sun, they are open during the day and closed at night. Like the sun, they are not contaminated by what they see. Speech arises out of breath and is intrinsically connected to it and hence to wind, but also to fire, because when the fire is gone from the body, speech departs. It also weakens when the fires of the stomach are not fed by food.[13] The mind has the qualities of the sky but is more often likened to the moon, for the mind waxes and wanes and is thus fickle. The quarters are the ears because both carry or hold sound, and the voice is the thunder from the heavens.

In a body construction that parallels the Upanishadic image of an assemblage of the various deities and elements, the later medieval *puranas* describe the creation of a body from the different qualities of several gods. In one myth the goddess Devi is created in parts by the energies of the other gods: her arms from one god, her face from another. Her emotions include the anger of the principal gods Vishnu and Shiva, and therefore she is more powerful and more dangerous than all the gods and demons.[14] The body is also visualized as made up of interchangeable parts, and sometimes these parts may be traded with animals. Ganesha is a deity with an elephant's head transplanted onto him by his father Shiva, who had himself cut off the son's head in rage.

In ancient Hindu thought the body is easily separable from the spirit, and many yogic practices are aimed at such a separation. On the other hand, this tendency of the body and spirit to split makes for vulnerability. A person can lose his or her soul and be relocated in other things and people, as the body can be penetrated by the spirits and other souls. The body can be possessed in love or by a god, and the soul itself can be split into parts.

SPEECH

In the hierarchy of body parts and functions, speech is next to *prana* and is naturally and explicitly associated with breath. Speech was Prajapati's first creation as he divided himself in two. From the union of these rest of the universe was created. The power of speech was recognized from the very beginning, because speech was the first instrument of sociality.[15]

For people in an oral culture, the spoken word was immensely important. The Vedic literature was *shruti*, meaning it was heard.[16] The *Sama Veda* and the Upanishads connected to it extol the virtues of speech, specifically the utterance of the syllable *Om,* and generally the rhythmic chanting of verse formulations, the *mantras. Om*—highest in the order of spoken words, indeed the original reverberation still resounding through the cosmos—gave to the *mantras* a primordial power with which the worshippers invoked their gods. The poets were conscious even at this time that the gods loved praise, and speech was a conduit to them. In the Vedic pantheon, each god was individually propitiated wih exaggerated praise; each in turn was celebrated as absolute, superior to all others. The *Chandogya Upanishad* says that people are dependent on praise, and love it as they do being a celebrity.[17] Hindus evince constant awareness of what their ancestors knew and formulated; they are quick to understand vainglory and a need for accolades. As words can enhance self-esteem, so can they hurt. As the Gujarati proverb goes, "Wounds from physical hurts heal, but those made by words never do." This is the reverse of the American saying "Sticks and stones may break my bones, but names will never hurt me."

FOOD

Food occupies an eminent place in an understanding of the body. In the *Aitareya Upanishad,* a sage declares that earth is "both food and consumer. [The worshipper] is both consumer and consumed. No one possesses that which he does not eat, or the things which do not eat him."[18] In the *Chandogya Upanishad* we see that the various properties of the body are connected to each other and that the three elements (earth, water, and fire) are contained in food.[19]

The *Taittiriya Upanishad* echoes the same spirit. "From food are produced all creatures which dwell on earth. They live by food, and in the end return to food. For food is the oldest of all beings and therefore it is called panacea."[20] It also declares that a man should never shun food.

The Hindu custom of not leaving home without eating, or symbolically touching food to one's mouth if at the time of departure food is mentioned, may well arise from such ancient injunctions. The same custom has it that one does not mention food or suggest eating when someone is leaving. In the same spirit, a person, even a stranger, is not to be turned away hungry— especially if he asks for food. "Let him never turn away (a stranger) from his house, that is the rule. Therefore a man should by all means acquire much food, for (good) people say (to the stranger) 'There is food ready for him.' If he gives food amply, food is given to him amply."[21]

In India, a universally practiced method of communicating anger and hurt feelings is to refuse food, and usually to refuse to talk as well. The Upanishadic poets saw refusal or inability to eat as a sign of sorrow. Announcing one's hurt through the practice of refusing food must arise from the awareness that when people are depressed and filled with sadness they cannot eat, and also from the Indian view that to refuse food, especially when offered, is an offense.[22] The hunger strikes of Mahatma Gandhi were not just self-purification but also a way of communicating anger and hurt, and the original offender was required to apologize and otherwise correct the wrong. Fasting is an established form of penance, a way of appeasing the gods, but also an effort to alter the behavior of the gods in a way pleasing to the worshipper.

Foods lend themselves to another classification according to the effects they have on the body. Yogis, students, and those conducting worship are required to eat substances that will not excite the body but calm it. These are *sattvika* foods, full of the qualities of light and purity.

The connection between breath and food is often repeated. It is clear that the people of the Upanishadic era must have concluded that the two were essential to the sustenance of life.

SAMKHYA

Samkhya is regarded as one of the oldest schools of Hindu thought and may have existed in India among the people before the arrival of the Indo-Europeans.[23] It postulates the primacy of matter and self. Because the medical enterprise begins with the idea of a misery-prone body and mind and has the removal of misery as its primary objective, *samkhya* offers yet another rationale to the medical physicians and metaphysicians.

Prakriti and *purusha,* the principles of materiality and consciousness, are the primordial entities of *samkhya.* Materiality is without consciousness but has the potential for activity. Consciousness is inactive, but when in proximity with materiality it makes the unmanifest manifest. It is presumed that the two are always in contact with each other, but consciousness is dependent on materiality for its eventual emancipation from the unstable world of activity and change. While the postulates of the system leave some questions about how inactive consciousness could activate matter in its nonsentient state, implicit in it is the idea of purposiveness.[24] An analogy is the relationship between a blind man who cannot see but can act and a lame one who can see but cannot move. The *samkhya* ideas of creation are clearly an attempt at distinguishing between the subjective and the objective, and the separate status given to materiality clearly makes it suitable for medical theory.

From the initial contact between materiality and consciousness emerges intelligence. This entity is also characterized by the three qualities (*gunas*), but light or spirit (*sattva*) is preponderant. Next comes the development of self-consciousness, *ahamkara*. Its principal characteristic is desire, a state of awareness which is clouded by the trappings of materiality, from which are differentiated the five subtle bodily substances and the objects of sensory organs: the word, touch, color (and form), taste, and smell. These seven together—intelligence, self-consciousness, and the five subtle substances— evolve from disturbances in materiality and have the potential for further transformation. Evolution now brings forth the five sensory organs, corre- sponding to the five bodily substances (the organs of hearing, touch, sight, taste, and smell) and the five organs of activity (of speech, touch, reproduc- tion, evacuation, and locomotion). The final and eleventh organ is *manas*, the faculty of apprehension and emotionality. The five *mahabhutas* (space, wind, fire, water, and earth) are added, and thus the body consists of twenty-four elements (including the original form of matter). The twenty-fifth is *purusha*, described as the prisoner of the body in the *Bhavaprakasha*, and now called the *atman* or *jivatman*.[25]

In *samkhya* thought, pain or disorder is of three types: intrinsic, extrinsic, and divine. This classification of pain corresponds to the Ayurvedic definition of diseases as endogenous, exogenous, and that which arises as a result of *karma*.[26] The humoral theory was also an aspect of *samkhya* thought, as were the Ayurvedic therapeutics. Moral conduct was important in avoidance of pain caused by external and superhuman forces.

If the *samkhya*-informed distinctions between consciousness and mate- riality are equivocally articulated in the Ayurvedic literature, the theory of intrinsic properties of substances may be regarded as the most profound influence of that school of medical thought. In all material things there are the three properties: goodness, vitality, and inertia. These are not abstract qualities; they are material and present in all matter. Food, colors, tastes, activities, and bodily substances are regarded as having a preponderance of one of the qualities.[27]

The three qualities have a variety of meaning in different contexts. On the physical plane *sattva* is cool and light, *rajas* is active and hot, and *tamas* is heavy and dull. At the psychological level, they are calm, passionate, and stupid or lethargic respectively. On the ethical plane the three are pure and virtuous, happy or sorrowful, and dark and evil and among colors white, red, and gray or black respectively. Contemplation, meditation, and devotion promote goodness. Love, battle, pleasure-seeking, and emotionality charac- terize vitality, and sloth, sleep, and idleness increase inertia. Among the body substances semen, blood, and fat epitomize the three *gunas* respectively.

Another important distinction emerging in *samkhya* is between a gross body and a subtle body. The gross body corresponds to the five created elements, while the subtle body includes intelligence, mind, and the ego-self. The physical and gross body perishes at death, while the subtle body accompanies the *atman* after death. The subtle body is unable to experience pleasure or pain without the gross body; it migrates from one body to another through rebirths until the person merges with *brahman*. The subtle body is atomic in size and is also the reservoir of a karmic record of actions.

YOGIC IMAGES

The Upanishads later emphasized by the stream of philosophic thought known as yoga put forth other images of the body. Although the physical health practices of yoga are well known in the West and its principles have been used in modern psychology (in meditation practices and biofeedback, for example), the foundations of yogic philosophy are integral to our understanding of the body imagery within this school of thought.

The *Yogasutra* of Patanjali, regarded as the most authentic early work on the subject, is usually dated around 200 B.C.E. This date for the compendium does not, however, reflect the antiquity of the theory and practice. From the evidence available to archeologists it has been argued that yoga was indigenous to India and was incorporated into Aryan and later Hindu thought.

The word *yoga* is derived from the Sanskrit root *yuj*, meaning "to bring together, to be in conjunction with," and is cognate with the English *yoke* and *join*. The object of yoga, Patanjali declares, is to prevent or inhibit the natural tendencies of the mind and to unite them in one-pointedness.[28] The theory also implies a regulation of body parts and their functions which would permit a person to concentrate and meditate. Thus later developments involved many elaborations depending on what aspect of body and mind was emphasized.

In the classical tradition the yogin is to withdraw his attention from the objects of sense-perception, avoid responding to internal or external stimuli, and attain a state of consciousness different from ordinary experience anchored in the world of objects. The stages of this practice lead ultimately to *samadhi,* in which the split between the phenomenal and the spiritual is obliterated. The organ of perception (*chitta*) perceives nothing, and the consciousness is thus liberated from dimensions of psychophysiological and temporal realities.[29]

In yogic thought, the layers of the body were visualized in an increasing order of priority of functions. These proceeded from the outside to the inside, from the grosser to the more subtle, from the harder to the softer, from the less vital to the more vital, from the material to the less material. Writers often compare this image of the person to an onion's concentric layers.

In the *Taittiriya Upanishad,* food forms the outermost layer of the body. The second layer consists of breath, and inhalation, exhalation, and the period between inhalation and exhalation are its parts. Next comes the layer of the mind, and various Vedic treatises are named as its parts. Within the layer of the mind is the layer of understanding. Faith is its head, knowing right from wrong and true from false are its limbs, and meditation is grounded in its organs of discrimination. The innermost layer is that of bliss, and its joy and satisfaction are grounded in *brahman.*[30]

An alternative concept of the body is seen in the *kundalini yoga* traditions. The spine is a vertical axis, along which are *chakras* (wheels or lotuses), which act as centers of energy and instinctual impulse. It is believed that the *kundalini,* the spiritual aspect of the person, lies sleeping in the lowest *chakra,* at the base of the spine. This spirituality must be awakened by special exercises and travel to the top of the head, to unite with Shiva, the principle of ultimate consciousness.

Here again the breath is invoked, for the *chakras* are centers of breath-energy and cannot be perceived by the senses. From these come the yogic nerves, the *nadis,* which are subtle channels for the currents of *prana.* The four *chakras* above the lowest are associated with genito-excretory, digestive, cardiac, and respiratory functions, while the higher ones are associated with thought and emotion. *Kundalini yoga* seeks to change the direction of flow in the nerves, gain control over the body's physical systems, and penetrate through thought and emotion to the source of individual energy and will. Most *kundalini* exercises involve some control of the breath. Many of these concepts are contained in the so-called yogic Upanishads (the most important are the *Yogatattva,* the *Dhyanabindu,* and the *Nadabindu*).

Parallel to the idea of the energy of breath traveling upward along the spinal axes is the idea that the semen retained by the yogin also travels upward. This semen is transformed by yogic practice into a source of physical, mental, and spiritual energy and stored in the brain.

In yogic thought the body becomes an obstacle to self-realization: instinctual impulses lead the person to focus upon material objects of pleasure, and these detract from concentration on the inner self-principle. In the discipline of *hatha yoga,* one of the several schools of thought that have emerged, elaborate physical postures are developed to gain control over the body and the pain that may arise from it.[31]

The idea of the discreteness of the body parts and their distinct origins has important implications for medicine. The discrete parts retain their autonomy and must therefore be united as a cohesive whole. The self performs these functions, and in the eyes of the Upanishadic poets, the wind is often the greatest uniter. The wind travels all over the body and regulates body functions, besides defining life itself.

Two kinds of selves emerged in Hindu thought, a transcendental and a phenomenal, but the former as a nonparticipating observer could not perform the function of uniting the body parts. The phenomenal self was therefore the natural agent of that function. The phenomenal self (and the phenomena themselves) had come to be equated with transience and hence with a false sense of I-ness; it needed to be shed to achieve spiritual authenticity. Thus the unity of body parts became precarious, unable to rely on the true and lasting self (which was beyond the measurable) and the phenomenal (which was fragile).

The vulnerable integrity and cohesiveness of the body are especially difficult to maintain in conditions of pain or illness. Body parts loosen their connections with each other and impinge on human consciousness as disconnected and noxious. Such a body construction helps explain the fact that body and body-parts consciousness, hypochondriacal preoccupations, and psychosomatic illnesses are encountered in Indian populations with higher frequencies.

If the cosmic giant Prajapati divided into various body parts out of a desire to propagate himself, so do humans when they become expansive, puffed up with pride. Desire splits selves apart, and they depend on a source outside themselves to become cohesive. The ego-self, *ahamkara*, constantly needs bolstering, and the body parts dependent on this weak agent for their unity are experienced with heightened consciousness. The body and its parts thus become the idiom of personal distress. On the other hand, a balance and harmony between the body constituents is the basis of good health.

·6·

Sexuality

Bloodshot from a sleepless night of passion, listless now
Your eyes express the mood of awakened love,
Damn you, Madhava! Go, Kesava, leave me!
Don't plead your lies with me!

Jayadeva, *Gitagovinda*

On the sidewalks of an Indian city one often finds a display of books, old and new, and set aside in one corner are books covered in yellow cellophane. These are modern versions and translations of what is collectively known as *kokashastra*. Nearby is a display of herbal drugs, roots, animal skin and horns, extracts, and so on. An itinerant pharmacist draws a crowd of people as he hawks these preparations, addressing universal concerns about aging and the loss of vitality. His supply of herbs grown in distant mountains holds hope for men whose sexual vigor is waning or for those who find their women unresponsive to their advances. Extravagant claims are made for these medicines: they give untiring erections, lure back estranged lovers and wives, cure women led astray by their hypersexuality. Such claims echo the concerns of a populace who fears loss of vigor and damage to sexual organs (especially to the quality of semen) from overindulgence. The sales techniques of the pharmacist reflect the cultural undercurrent of concern with sexuality that is clearly apparent in Hindu medical texts and sex manuals.

PLEASURE, PASSION, AND RESTRAINT

Kama, sensual pleasure, is one of the four aims of Hindu life; it is celebrated in the ancient and medieval literature collectively called *kamashastra*. The third-century *Kamasutra* of Vatsayana, the earliest surviving treatise on love and sex, is the principal text.[1]

Kama is also the name of the Hindu god of love, who affects humans and gods alike with no regard for traditional boundaries. He is also called Ananga, "without a body," because his body was burnt to ashes by the wrath

58

of Shiva (whom he aroused from a deep state of meditation by stimulating Shiva's passions). The other gods had asked Kama to rouse Shiva so he would notice his wife and produce a son; the son had been prophesied as the slayer of a demon terrorizing the gods.

The *Kamasutra* deals with an upper-class man-about-town and his mistress, who lead lives of hedonistic delight. A wide variety of carnal pleasures are legitimized: prostitution, adultery, group sex, homosexuality, biting and making nail marks to increase sexual pleasure, and aphrodisiacs. Woman equals man in capacity for sexual pleasure, and the secret of masculine success is in bringing a woman to full coital pleasure. The *Kamasutra* has advice for acquiring and then courting a wife, showing how to win her confidence and introduce her to love.

The love manuals are not exempt from the Hindu fascination with classification: the *Kamasutra* provides details on coital postures and sets out levels of passion according to types of women. Men and women are advised how to retain the love of a spouse or friend. The tone of the *Kamasutra* is matter-of-fact, and sexual impulses are treated as natural but often overwhelming.

In another arena of discourse, however, fear of women's sexuality had emerged. Intercourse with sexually mature women was thought to result in the loss of youth and vigor. Both folklore and texts on sex advocated union with young and virginal women for men seeking sexual rejuvenation. Men and women were categorized according to the size of their genitalia and degrees of passion. The rise and fall of passions were also connected to the movements of the stars, the phases of the moon, the seasons. Astrological charts were used to predict sexual passion and behavior. Sexual dysfunctions including lack of desire, inability to perform, premature ejaculation, and loss of beauty and vitality were matters of literate as well as popular discourse. The later texts on sexuality can be understood better as manuals on sex therapy than as advocates of the "joy of sex."

The twelfth-century *Kokashastra* and the sixteenth-century *Ananga Ranga* capture this changing ethos. Free and easy sexuality is replaced with warnings against adultery. The ostensible purpose of the texts is to enhance marital bliss by laying down rules for virtuous women. A woman is to be chaste and to serve her husband as a god, a prized possession, and a source of happiness.

In the *kama* texts, the body is portrayed as a group of constituent parts, each a center for enjoyment. This is in keeping with body construction in the earlier texts. In the *Ananga Ranga* the locus of sexuality shifts to various body parts according to the phases of the moon.

A passage from the *Mahabharata* (400 B.C.E.–400 C.E.) is often cited to contrast an earlier period of free sexuality with the conservative ethic of the later period. King Pandu, who was childless because of a curse, explains to his wife Kunti the origins of proper sexual conduct: "In the olden days, so we hear, the women were uncloistered, they were their own mistresses who took their pleasure where it pleased them. From childhood on they were faithless to their husbands, but yet not lawless, for such was the law in olden days."[2]

According to the *Mahabharata* the law that "favored women" was later changed by Svetaketu, the son of a great seer. His mother was taken away in full view of Svetaketu and his father when a brahmin simply suggested that she go with him. The son became enraged at this insult, but the father calmed him by invoking the eternal law: "Just as the cows do, so do the creatures each in its class."[3] But Svetaketu, finding this acceptable for animals but not for humans, laid down a new law: "From this day on, a woman's faithlessness to her husband shall be a sin equal to aborticide, an evil that shall bring on misery. Seducing a chaste woman and a constant wife who is avowed to her husband shall also be a sin on earth."[4]

The conservative turn in the Hindu attitude toward sexuality is the work of the lawgivers, the composers of *dharmashastra*. The Vedic texts, although exhibiting unmistakable patriarchalism, were open in their regard for natural body functions, body parts, and sexual relationship. The Vedic gods had consorts, and Indra was known particularly as a seducer of women. Sexual union was a prime model of creation and creativity. When Prajapati split himself into two, it was because he could not experience delight in being alone, and he had a desire to propagate himself. In the Vedic period sexuality was associated not only with fertility but also with pleasure, a legitimate craving. On the other hand, the lawgivers (Manu is an excellent example) became most concerned with the householder's need for a wife. They imagined the female sexual power, the fire in a woman's body, as not easily calmed. Regulation of her sexuality became an important objective of social custom and moral law, thus permitting the determination of paternity and the lines of inheritance.

Increasing social stratification included rules of endogamy. These rules also decreed that the sexuality of men, but more particularly of women, be contained within the confines of marriage to secure the purity of caste groups. We may infer that the development of ascetic practices like yoga were also responsible for turning sexuality into a distracting influence. Woman was associated with both matter and illusion, both of which kept the yogin from enlightenment. Although pleasure (*kama*) was retained as a legitimate aim of life for the householder, there was a decisive turn away from indulgence of the senses; the body and the bodily self were viewed as obstacles to realization of spiritual goals.

From the late medieval period until recently, successive invaders overthrew local chieftains and kings and established monarchies. Hindu society became increasingly conservative and closed. The Muslims introduced *purdah*, which kept women veiled and off the streets, and many Hindus followed that custom. Muslims dominated India from the thirteenth century C.E. until the entrance of the British in the second half of the eighteenth century, who brought with them Victorian cultural ideals and restrictions on sexual freedom.

Love (*shringara*) is one of the nine cardinal emotions in Hindu drama and psychology, and one of the most important. Love between gods and goddesses has inspired both ancient and modern poetry. The *Kumarasambhavam* of Kalidasa celebrates the union of Shiva and Parvati, and its lurid description of their intercourse embarrasses college professors, I am told, who avoid these passages in their classrooms. The *Gitagovinda* of Jayadeva, a twelfth-century work, concentrates on the passionate love of Krishna and the cowherdess Radha. Later devotional (*bhakti*) poetry all over India drew inspiration from this love poem. Krishna is the epitome of all lovers, and the Vaishnavas, his devotees, seek vicarious union with him through sexual imagery. Edward Dimock introduces his translations of *bhakti* poetry by observing that "most of the lyrics of the Bengal Vaishnavas are in the mood called *madhurya-bhava,* in which the poet is considering Krishna in his aspect of divine lover; he writes as if he himself were Radha or one of the Gopis [companions of Radha]."[5]

Separation and union are major themes of love poetry all over India. Even in the less religious and more ordinary love songs of the cinema, or in Urdu love poetry, the same pattern prevails. Lovesickness was a well-recognized problem, and the *Ananga Ranga* lists ten stages from fascination through insanity to death.[6]

MARRIAGE

Even today in India most brides and grooms are complete strangers to each other. Sexual intimacy in these circumstances is a ritual, but one full of apprehension and anticipation. The opportunity for privacy is limited after the initial period of marriage, during which the family provides isolation for the new couple. Later on when children share sleeping quarters with the parents, particularly with the mother, privacy is limited further. Sexual spontaneity between a married couple is often constrained. Most couples tend to have intercourse almost fully clothed. The couple may or may not grow to love each other, and the relationship may or may not go beyond the obligatory ritual transactions.

An Indian anthropologist, Veena Das, has accurately analyzed the restraint on sexuality within marriage. In contrasting the fulfillment of erotic desires and the obligation to procreate, she points out that the physical descriptions of semen itself provide a clue. The texts she cites suggest that from indulgence of passions semen becomes watery, while a man pursuing the marital obligation to procreate has semen with the qualities of molten silver and the smell of lotuses. The treatment of coitus within marriage as a ritual act means that semen is regarded as pure, unlike other products of the body.[7]

From patients and other informants I have learned that the constraints on marital sexuality cause psychological anxieties. Anxieties of clinical proportion result in sexual dysfunctions. Given the Indian emphases on containment of semen and passion, the most common dysfunction among men is premature ejaculation. Another common problem is "leakage." Morris Carstairs, a Scottish psychiatrist, describes a syndrome in which the male patient complains that he is losing semen involuntarily in his urine, that his body is being sapped of energy and vitality. Gananath Obeyesekere, an anthropologist, expands the notion, considering women who regard a whitish vaginal discharge (leucorrhea) as a loss of body substance.[8] In Gujarat, women suffering from the condition speak of their "bodies being washed away."

In a culture that stresses the body's construction out of autonomous and discrete parts, vulnerability to incoherence is heightened. Powerful and at times uncontainable sexual impulses exaggerate the concentration on genitalia, disconnecting them from the total or whole being. As the mother of a grown daughter expressing reluctance to get married in face of several "offers" said, "Your mind may not want to, but your body will." On a spectrum from the normal to the pathological, this mind/body split prevails among most Hindus, resulting in compulsive sexuality in some at the pathological end. These attitudes contribute to the difficulty in narrowing the aims of sexuality to a particular person, when the satisfaction of the body part rather than the person is a pressing need. Furthermore, the diffusion of sexual aim leads to mild suspicion or frank distrust in matters of fidelity, which surfaces often as a theme in Hindu literature.[9]

TANTRA AND SALVATION

Tantra, among the more peripheral sects in India, is notorious both in India and in the West for its esoteric sexual practices. The awe of feminine powers is an essential aspect of this ritualistic form of worship. *Tantra* means to broaden and extend knowledge. One way it does so is by incorporating the female substance into the male body. In an attempt to gain the upper hand in relation to the woman, while ultimately denying the need for her, some tantric practitioners find bliss by reversing the flow of substances from male to female, first by a retrograde ejaculation and then by attempting to absorb the female sexual fluids, using the urethra as a pipette.

This practice is designed to overcome the fear of women. The Bengali saint Ramakrishna Paramahamsa, who was a worshipper of the goddess Kali and practiced *tantra*, noted: "I am very much afraid of women. When I look at one, I feel as if a tigress were coming to devour me . . . [I] look upon them as she-monsters."[10] Ramakrishna also dressed as a woman and imagined himself as a woman to liberate himself from the power of attraction and repulsion women held for him. He sought to transfer his attraction for human women to Kali, to have his soul love intensely while his body was inert, like a piece of wood or stone.

Kundalini yoga, an extension of the tantric tradition, describes the goddess at the bottom of a person's spine as a curled snake. She climbs the spine to unite with her lover Shiva, who rests in the lotus at the top of the head. Here the union of male and female brings liberation.

Gods too may take on female forms. As Shiva states to the Devi in the *Devi Bhagavata*: "Now that I have got this youthful feminine form before thee, there is not a trace of desire within me to get again my masculine form."[11]

Sudhir Kakar, an Indian psychoanalyst, points out that *tantra* has "always provided a cultic home for many types of deviants from Hindu orthodoxy, as well as those who, because of their lower caste or their sex, could not fully participate in the Brahminical system." According to Kakar, *tantra* professes the equality of men and women and allows women to be tantric, but the main thrust of the tradition is for males to achieve "the realization of both masculinity and femininity within the tantrik's own body, the experience of a constant, doubled joy of 'two-in-one,' the recreation of primordial androgyny."[12]

Tantra envisions three stages of development. The first stage, in which traditional morality is accepted, is an animal existence. The next stage is that of the hero who conquers the fears of sexuality and death, violates traditional morality, and conquers the mother-goddess or becomes her slave. Finally in the divine form the practitioner transcends traditional morality to a state in which all objects have equal value.

The aspect of *tantra* that involves the equation of sex with death has not been sufficiently appreciated. In that sense the tantric returns to the earlier Hindu preoccupation with overcoming death. At a more mundane level, the loss of semen and erection after an orgastic ejaculation is the basis of the comparison. At the ritual level is corpse meditation, through which one conquers the fear of death. The practitioner sits on a corpse's back at night and calls in the mother-goddess to inhabit the corpse and save him from the ghosts and demons of the cremation grounds. When the corpse is "awakened," the tantric realizes either detachment from death or dependence on the Mother (Kali).

One sexual ritual of devotion to the Mother uses a mistress or prostitute to gain power over the Mother. The practitioner uses chants during the ritual coitus, worships the deity in the *yoni* (vagina), becomes absorbed in the great enchantress, and thus conquers the fear of loss and impurity.[13]

What has not been emphasized in the foregoing discussion is the essential religious mantle of tantric practice. All is done in pursuit of unity with the mother-goddess, who in Hindu iconography dances over the body of Shiva. Shiva's image as an ascetic and a perpetual lover (his representation is the *lingam*, the phallus) with an ever-erect penis conveys the idea of an all-powerful ascetic, the only one who can conquer the ever-lustful female. Tantric sexuality is a religious practice leading not to offspring but to salvation.

THE BEGINNING OF LIFE

For an understanding of the process of conception we must turn to Ayurveda. The question of when life begins is not explicitly raised, but there are many discussions on the formation of an embryo after the mixing of male semen and female "blood." Medical texts provide instruction for the sexual union, following the same pattern as the scriptures.

When does life begin, and how? The *Carakasamhita* answers in the form of a debate.[14] It suggests that an embryo is formed by the union of the mother, the father, the life principle, an appropriateness of context (time, mood, suitability of partners), nourishment, and the principle of consciousness, and that none of these factors is capable of producing an embryo independently. In this dialogue, it is evident that Hindu medicine regards the beginning of life as the moment of conception. Not only is the embryo endowed at conception with the properties it receives from both the parents at a moment of appropriateness, but the life principle enters the process. With good nourishment the embryo develops in due course into a fetus and after birth through all the stages of life.

The sixteenth-century *Bhavaprakasha* presents a similar argument that life begins at conception. The properties of the self or the life principle remain the same: the *jivatma* is responsible for such qualities as desire, misery, happiness, effort, intelligence, and blinking of the eyes. Although the medical systems seem to have viewed the self as without properties, frequently they seem to return to an early Upanishadic view that equates the principle of self with breathing and consciousness.[15] Later, the same *atman*, or self, is presented as the precursor of knowing, misery, and happiness. The commentator asserts that we must interpret this to mean that proximity to the propertyless *atman*, and not *atman* itself, is the cause of these three characteristics.[16] This relatively late text differs from the *Carakasamhita* in its assumption that the principle of life is not extrinsic in semen or the uterine "blood." It uses the analogy of a magnifying glass and the rays of the sun, neither of which have overt fire in them. Yet when they come into a correct conjunction, the fire inherent in them becomes manifest. The text asserts that the unfolding of the life principle in the male and female germs when they combine with each other occurs in a similar way.[17]

The assumption is that the origin of a person and his body parts is in the "semen and blood" of the father and mother respectively. The texts offer an embryology with attention to every body part. Generally, that which is soft is posited as having arisen from the mother, and that which is hard from the father. Thus body hair, bones, nails, teeth, tendons, nerves, arteries, semen, and other firm parts come from the father, and flesh, blood, fat, marrow, heart, umbilicus, liver, spleen, intestines, and other soft parts come from the mother.

The authors go to great lengths to explain fetal and congenital abnormalities as products of defective male or female seeds, unnatural coitus, or weakness in one or more of the three humors (*doshas*). Miscarriage, stillbirth, and multiple pregnancy are explained in this paradigm. The growth of the fetus is attributed to the mother's nutrition, which is particularly emphasized.[18] A woman's mental state and circumstances are also implicated in the qualities of an unborn child. Childlessness is explained as failure of all the necessary conditions to come together, and determination of gender in terms of the preponderance of the male or the female seed.[19]

These germinal ideas find their way into the life of modern Hindus. Conception, pregnancy, and birth are an unfolding of the mystery of life. Anthropologists Ronald Inden and Ralph Nicholas attest to Bengali beliefs about conception rooted in Ayurvedic formulations.[20] Childless couples eat foods considered to increase generative substances, pregnant women are cared for with special recognition that their physical and mental states will determine the quality of the unborn child, and the postpartum care of baby and mother proceed according to principles laid down in the ancient texts.

The tensions, rituals, beliefs, and practices surrounding the events from conception to birth demonstrate a continuity of ancient and modern ways.

Pregnancy is an occasion for great joy, and the anticipation of a son heightens the eagerness of the entire family. The pregnant woman (especially during the first pregnancy) experiences an immediate change in her status. She is now the instrument of generational continuity.

SURROGATE MOTHERHOOD AND ARTIFICIAL INSEMINATION

An organized body of knowledge for the ethical resolution of conflicts inherent in modern medicine is yet to be formulated in India. Given the diversity of belief and practice this task is overwhelming. But in the day-to-day life of Hindus, folk history is an important source of inspiration and moral examples. Ancient myths are renewed and reshaped, and as in the Hindu use of history, they become answers to philosophical and psychosocial dilemmas. It cannot be overemphasized that without an authoritative book or prophet to interpret ethical conduct for all Hindus at different times, the mythologies of ancestors serve as examples, and a single proper course does not exist.

When a new conflict presents itself, people make up a code of conduct by searching ancient lore for an appropriate example. When contraception became an issue, for example, public discussion concentrated on whether the practice was known to Indian forebears. Abortion was legalized after legislative debates, and public argument was carried out mainly in secular newspapers and professional journals that borrowed heavily from ancient texts, both medical and religious, for supporting and opposing arguments. The major opposition came from the Christian minority in India. We must remember that with illiteracy in the range of 60 to 75 percent even these debates were not accessible to the multitudes, which usually resort to minstrels, narrators of mythology, and folk theaters for the interpretation of such problems.

In treating bioethical issues (like those surrounding surrogacy and artificial insemination), I have tried therefore to find in scriptural and medical texts the instances that might be adduced to resolve newly emerging conflicts.

In the *Mahabharata* the birth of the heirs to the Kuru kingdom, Dhritarashtra and Pandu, follows a classic pattern. The young son of the king was not able to produce offspring and died childless; the lineage was threatened with extinction. In such a moment of distress a different law was thought to apply. The mother of the dead king had a son born to her before her marriage. That son was called upon by law to impregnate the dead king's wives. Thus were born Dhritarashtra and Pandu. This kind of sexual union, called *niyoga*, is known in India today.[21]

Niyoga was the appointment by law of a man to cohabit with a woman for the purpose of producing a son. The appointment was sought when a man died without a son or was unable to have one because of a disability. The most appropriate person for the appointment was the husband's brother, failing which someone from the same lineage or caste could be chosen. A brahmin, considered to be a desirable father, might also be chosen. The sexual union by such an ordinance was to be accomplished without lust, as a duty, with permission of elders, and only once during the menstrual cycle until a son was produced. The son belonged to the woman's legal husband. The woman was the field and the husband the owner of the field, the appointed man merely the sower of the seed.

The childless Kunti, wife of Pandu, was encouraged and persuaded by her husband to have sons for him by invoking the law laid down by Svetaketu: "And a wife who is enjoined by her husband to conceive a child and refuses shall incur the same evil" (equal to abortion); and "Therefore, on seeing all these good reasons, you must without blame do my word, which obeys the law."[22] Pandu goes on to urge his wife to sleep with a "brahmin of superior austerity" and to have sons because the law decrees that she must give him sons. She had been granted a boon, which she then invoked to have the gods cohabit with her. She had three sons in this manner (another son had been born before her marriage, when she had inadvertently invoked one of the gods).

There are other means of conception in the *Mahabharata*. One is of particular significance in the context of modern technology. The birth of the sons of the blind king Dhritarashtra and his wife Gandhari seem almost a science-fiction story, for the embryonic development occurs in pots not unlike test tubes.

Gandhari had been granted a boon by the sage Vyasa and had asked for a hundred sons. She conceived but for two years failed to give birth to the fetus. "And when she felt the hardness of her own belly she began to worry . . . (and) fainting with pain, aborted her belly with hard effort. A mass of flesh came forth, like a dense ball of clotted blood." Vyasa, "best of the mumblers of spells," reappeared. To fulfill the boon he had granted Gandhari, he asked that a hundred pots be set up and filled with ghee," and he sprinkled the ball with cold water. "When the ball was doused it fell apart into a hundred pieces, each an embryo the size of a thumb joint; a full one hundred and one duly developed. . . . He put them in pots and had them watched in well-guarded places." In time a hundred sons and a daughter were born.[23]

A myth like this could be advanced to show the ethical acceptability of test-tube babies for Hindus. Similarly, a case could be made for ovum donation and the implantation of a fertilized ovum. The desire for offspring is strong, and fertility is sought through a variety of means. I myself encountered in a clinical situation a couple's attempt to conceive a child by having the wife sleep with the husband's friend. Infertility is a major source of stress, especially for women, who bear the brunt of the social stigma and psychological strife.

Another myth about conception and pregnancy allows us to construct a case for surrogacy. Several variations of the story of the birth of Krishna and his brother Balarama may guide the resolution of modern dilemmas concerning reproduction. King Kamsa was warned that the eighth child of his sister Devaki and Vasudeva would slay him. The king imprisoned the couple and killed the first six of their children. The seventh was saved by a goddess's intervention: the embryo was removed from the womb of Devaki and implanted in the womb of Vasudeva's other wife. The eighth child, Krishna himself, was saved by an exchange with another newborn who was later killed by the evil king. This is an important part of the legend of Krishna and appears in various *puranas*.[24]

A similar account surrounds the birth of the last liberated sage in the Jain religion of India. Mahavira descended from his divine place as an embryo in the womb of a poor brahmin woman. Dissatisfied with the family into which the sage would be born, the god Indra transferred the embryo into the womb of a woman in the caste of rulers and warriors (*kshatriya*), exchanging it for the one that was in her womb. Such exchanges were generally performed by the gods.[25]

ABORTION AND INFANTICIDE

Abortion is a more complicated matter, and the gap between theory and practice cannot be overemphasized. Hindu rules of conduct derive legitimacy from and are enforced through the institutions of family and caste, not organized religion. Commenting on Hindu attitudes, demographer Sripati Chandrasekhar states: "as in all codes of ethics, there is in the Hindu view an admirable and practical dichotomy of the ideal and the permissible. The ideal code of behavior was for the dedicated 'righteous' or saintly minority and the permissible way was for the work-a-day million."[26]

The early texts consider abortion to be a sin equal to the killing of a learned person. *Bhruna-hatya,* the killing of a fetus, is a word also used for the murder of a brahmin. The practice was condemned in the *Atharva Veda,* one of the four revealed sources of knowledge, as well as in the later *smriti* literature. The fifth-century *Yagnavalkya Smriti* states: "The undoubted degradation of women is caused by sexual intercourse with the lowly-born, causing abortion (in oneself) and causing injury to the husband." The same *smriti* considers induced abortion as grounds for abandoning one's wife.[27]

Medical texts like the *Sushrutasamhita* describe ways of destroying a fetus in cases of fetal death or obstructed labor. Acharya Lolimbaraja, a seventeenth-century Ayurvedic physician, advises that "if the root of the herb *Indrayam* is kept in the vagina, menstrual discharge begins. It is a useful remedy for pregnant women in poor health, widows and women of liberal morals."[28]

Abortion has been legal in India since 1972. The act did not create much religious controversy, nor has there been any significant drop in birth rates since its implementation. Its effectiveness as a population control measure is negligible. Experts point out that unchecked population growth, which is the most critical health problem in India, cannot be tackled by abortions or even sterilizations. In their view the solution lies in the education of women, better and more accessible health care especially for infants, and a general improvement in the standard of living. The major beneficiaries of legalized abortion are women who conceive out of wedlock, for whom the pregnancy is a matter of social stigma.

In the modern era one technological advance that raises significant concerns is amniocentesis. In a culture where sons are overwhelmingly favored, the availability of a method of sex determination is bound to cause a stir. Neglect of female babies and female infanticide in India is neither a new nor a negligible problem.[29]

Amniocentesis, though not yet widely or cheaply available, shifts the focus to infanticide in the prenatal period. Activists for women's rights are very concerned about this development. Legalized abortion has been an important gain, according to them, for those who wish to terminate pregnancy for whatever reason. But the overwhelming preference for sons when amniocentesis is freely available puts a female fetus at great risk. Moreover, neither physicians nor legislators have responded to their pleas for a ban on amniocentesis for the purpose of sex determination. They also point out that most social reform movements in India run against the established principles of tradition, and they have not found interpreters of traditional law to help them crusade against the use of amniocentesis for sex selection.[30]

ATTITUDES TOWARD WOMEN

It is difficult for moderns to grasp fully the devaluation of women in ancient times. Surely the Hindu situation appears no different in this regard from other civilizations of that time. Inequality between men and women, and particularly the domination of women by men, was an aspect of all early cultures. We may speculate that in the transformation of nomadic and pastoral life to a settled agriculture, men came to dominate women. In the process of this transformation family life developed within a social organization around the ownership of property (land and cattle); the family became the unit of a property-based economy. We may assume that over a long period—from the Vedic period to the time of the epics and the *puranas*—men became the leaders and patriarchs, formulating laws governing the modes of conduct of that social organization. Rules governing the transmission of property from generation to generation required that patrimony be fixed. In the *dharmashastra* literature, we find a curtain dropping on the freedom and equality of women, an overelaborate matrix of family lines, and an overemphasis on the male line of progeny. As we saw above, a variety of methods for obtaining a son were legitimized (some anticipating the methods of modern technology) in the effort to prolong the family line.

The Hindu scheme of male-female relationships was further complicated by the periodic "impurity" of women. Laws concerning purity and pollution provided a rationale for subordinating women as property rights became an issue in the evolution of an agricultural system. Education was another vehicle of male dominance, and men writing laws wrote in favor of themselves (as the brahmins did in their own favor).

A more far-reaching and speculative explanation may be found in the larger civilizational process. Damodar D. Kosambi, a mathematician, archeologist, and Sanskritist, has advanced a theory that the wars between the Aryans and the early inhabitants of India were a struggle between the patriarchy of the invaders and the matriarchy of the inhabitants, a process universal to early civilizations.[31] We may infer that unlike the encounters of the Greeks, Egyptians, and Mesopotamians with these rivals, in the Indian situation the patriarchal invaders never completely demolished the native matriarchal cultures. Hence ambivalent attitudes toward women, their social devaluation, and a psychological fear of them have persisted to the present.

In the *dharmashastra* literature the position of women oscillates. Often women are compared to the lowest caste (*shudras*), undeserving of Vedic training, respect, or admiration. As wives they are considered agents of strife—inferior, hypersexual, and wicked. As mothers they are exalted, seen as instruments of generational continuity and nurturers. Over time, their status diminished, and men sought means to control them. Male fear of female sexuality left women isolated in the domestic sphere. Daughters were seen as a burden to the father and the family.

Early marriages for women became the norm in India. To avoid the possibility of girls' experiencing sexual impulses and intercourse before marriage, fathers were required by law to give daughters away in marriage before puberty. Not arranging the marriage of a girl before her first menstrual period came to be regarded as a sin, and a daughter so neglected was permitted to choose her own mate three months after her menarche, according to an older *dharmasutra* text. The *Laws of Manu* extends that period to three years.[32] It is also possible that the menses was seen as a kind of abortion, or at least a wasted opportunity, for the texts hold the father responsible for the sin of destroying an embryo at each menses. In practice, prepubertal marriages for women were the norm in the villages of India, and tales of "cradle marriages" have also been reported.

The Sharada Act, also known as the Prevention of Child Marriages Act, was passed in 1929 and later amended to fix the minimum age of marriage at sixteen. This law has had some impact on child marriage, but the more important influences have been education, urban life, and modernization. The heroic efforts of female social reformers have given some relief from coercive marriage practices in urban areas, but reports of violations of the Sharada Act continue to flow in from villages.

In most parts of India the bride is considered a gift to the groom, and the lawgivers classified acceptable marriages by the amount of other material gifts. The dowry system is an outgrowth of this principle. In modern times the system has become notorious because of the "dowry death"—the unexpected death of a young bride, usually by murder and burning, because she did not bring enough in dowry or because the husband and his mother conspired to make possible a second marriage which would bring in another dowry. The mother-son relationship is intense, for the mother derives her special status and self-esteem from her son, and the situation of the bride is complicated by that dynamic. The young bride takes the son away from his mother and is really an intruder into their relationship. Hence she is subject to all manner of rejection and humiliation, and in some instances murder. In parts of India there is a high incidence of suicide among new brides.

The position of a young widow, especially a childless one, is the most pitiable. She is by tradition made a scapegoat for her husband's death and excluded from religious ceremonies. Until it became outlawed in 1829 under British rule, *sati*—self-immolation by widows on their husbands' funeral pyres—was common, especially in Rajasthan and Bengal. Ram Mohan Roy, the nineteenth-century Hindu reformist, led a social movement against this cruel custom. Arguments about how ancient the custom was and whether the Vedas required a widow to immolate herself were left largely unsettled. Roy, who had been influenced by the British, invoked values outside the Hindu tradition to turn Indians against *sati*.[33] An occurrence of *sati* in Rajasthan in September 1987 shocked the nation.

In later Hindu thought, sexual morality for men and women was complicated by the conviction that women were sexually uncontainable and were the cause of a man's physical decline. Women were mothers of beautiful sons and lifegiving mother-goddesses on one hand, and seductive, lustful, and wicked temptresses on the other. These dual attitudes surface repeatedly throughout Indian history. We may presume that the fertile and powerful mother-goddesses of the non-Aryans and their earthy rituals produced in the Hindus these mixed images. Negative attitudes about the sexuality of women are present in the *Laws of Manu* and the later *kama* texts. The expanding boundaries of the Hindu civilization and interaction with the dark-colored natives raised concerns about the mixing of races. In turn, rules in marriage, especially those concerning sexual conduct, became more conservative, with an emphasis on social control of female sexuality. This period may have begun after the time of the Buddha. *Brahmacharya,* conduct according to *brahman,* became a high virtue. Adherents took vows of celibacy, led austere lives, and devoted themselves to learning and yogic practices in search of self-realization. Distrust of women and their potential for being faithless to their husbands evolved into strict control and regulation of their conduct.

It is generally understood in India that sexual impulses need external controls, for internalized controls cannot exist. As a Gujarati proverb goes, "When you put *ghee* [clarified butter] on a hot plate, it melts." Parents take precautions against having young men and women meet in privacy. By the same logic, a man and a woman meeting privately are assumed to be sexually involved.

Often this attitude toward sexuality leads to a separation between romantic love and sexual love. The mechanics of intercourse become more important, and the act is reduced to mere physical pleasure. An Indian man once told me that what he craved was "spinal sex," a physical act not involving the brain or higher nervous system at all, and this attitude appears widespread among Indian men today. The union of mind, body, and emotion is needed to oppose such sexual alienation, which has its roots in a fragmented view of self and sexual expression.

·7·

Ayurveda: The Hindu Medical Tradition

*Health is known as happiness
while disorder is unhappiness.*
Carakasamhita

In Ayurvedic medicine illness is viewed simply as a state of imbalance. The physical, psychological, social, and spiritual realms are parts of the all-encompassing realm of Ayurveda. Illness and wellness are not mutually exclusive; circumstances and intentions determine the proportions of illness and wellness.

The Hindu world is best seen as a series of ever-widening circles extending into infinity. At the center is the private self. Each circle exerts an influence on the center in direct proportion to the size of the influencing object and in inverse proportion to its distance from the center. The kind and degree of illness may thus be visualized as a function of disturbance in any circle or in a combination of them. Given the complexity of Hindu society, the circles of influence do not assume fixed orbits.

The *Carakasamhita* speaks of *dhatusamya*, a balance of bodily substances, as a state of health. We may regard this ideal as a humoral balance that gives comfort and pleasure to mind, body, and senses. The *Sushrutasamhita*, in emphasizing the reciprocity of influences, regards not only the balance of humors but also the balance of physical, sensory, and mental dispositions as vital.[1]

In a system that changes with every kind of input and tends toward imbalance, remaining in a state of equilibrium is a tall order. There is hardly a state of disequilibrium of the humors in which the authors of Ayurvedic texts do not implicate anger, jealousy, excessive desire, laziness, and so on. By the same token, outside influences like dietetic input may alter psychological states.

73

For the average person, nothing is to be gained from suffering, and means are sought to alleviate pain and disease. Medical and ethical systems of thought seek to explain the antecedents of illness and offer remedies for cure and prevention. Only those who have renounced the pleasures of life (attachments, possessions, "I-ness," family, occupation, and so on) to embark on an ascetic way of life consciously subject their bodies to privation and pain. Others suffer, but involuntarily.

SOURCES, ASSUMPTIONS, AND PRINCIPLES

The corpus of Hindu literature pertaining to health and medicine is called Ayurveda, the science of vitality and long life. *Ayur,* meaning life, is the continuance of consciousness, animation, and the sustenance of the body.[2] As a Veda, these early writings are counted as sacred. It has been suggested that Ayurveda is a minor Veda, a supplemental or subsidiary limb, especially of the *Atharva Veda.* The *Atharva Veda* is considered to be the last of the four Vedas, the revealed literature. Nevertheless, its contents do not necessarily follow such a chronology. The text contains many prayers and chants to appease the gods but also mantras to ward off evil, misfortunes, diseases, and enemies. In contrast to the other Vedas, *Atharva Veda* resorts to magical explanations of the powers of unseen forces.

On the other hand, the *Atharva Veda* refers to itself as *Bhesaj Veda,* the Veda of medicinal plants.[3] The *atharvan* priests demonstrated their knowledge of the properties of plants and prescribed propitiatory rites, fasting and expiation.

The earlier Vedic texts of about 1500–1000 B.C.E. expressed concerns about the dread of afflictions and old age and prescribed cures involving prayers and a variety of plant products side by side. More important, the Ayurvedic construction of the body and its parts is continuous with the Vedic formulations. According to one Indologist, "In the Vedic texts we find the beginning of a science of anatomy, of an embryology and of a hygiene. In the *Satapatha Brahmana* (X and XII) and in the *Atharvaveda* (X, 2) we find an accurate enumeration of the bones of the human skeleton."[4]

The origin of medical knowledge is attributed in the Ayurvedic texts to a mixture of what is heard from divine sources and what is remembered from the teachings of sages. The *Carakasamhita,* the primary and the oldest known Ayurvedic text, opens with an assembly of sages. A sort of blue-ribbon committee, they had gathered at a retreat in the Himalayas because the populace was inflicted with diseases that interfered with the observances of religious obligations.[5] Desiring a disease-free state, the sages delegated

Bhardwaja to go to Indra, a god often identified with medicine and knowledgeable about cures (Indra had received instructions from the Ashwins, the heavenly physicians, who in turn had received the knowledge from the creator Brahma himself).[6] In the *Sushrutasamhita,* a text with a special emphasis on surgery, the source of knowledge is equally divine, with Dhanvantari as the intermediary sage. According to a later myth about the churning of the sea, Dhanvantari, another physician of the gods, had emerged from the ocean carrying *amrita,* the death-defying elixir. Later Ayurvedic texts repeat similar accounts of the origin of the medical sciences.

In the evolution and spread of medical knowledge and practice, Buddhist and later Jain scholars made vital contributions. Antibrahminical spirit permitted the Buddhist medical men to investigate, experiment, and break caste barriers freely (one interpretation holds that *carak,* or "itinerant," applied most aptly to Buddhist monks). At the early stages Buddhist thought was in many important respects a continuation of Hindu beliefs and practices and in turn influenced later Hindu thought and medicine.

The Ayurvedic texts place the medical tradition squarely within the larger province of traditional religious pursuits and philosophy. The survival of such accounts of the transmission of medical knowledge attests that medical theory and practice affected and were affected by the Hindu tradition.

The opening of the *Carakasamhita* asserts that a body free from disease is essential to the realization of life's tasks, including the spiritual. Ayurveda for the early physician was eternal knowledge created before the creation of the world. The potential for the protection of health and the removal of disorders was built into the act of creation. Health-seeking was a religious obligation, and traditional prescriptions were medicinal ones.

The Ayurvedic worldview is based on Hindu conceptions of humanity in relation to the universe and has endured over centuries, continuing both to inform and limit the health expectations of patients and the healing practices of physicians. Physicians schooled in allopathic medicine are forced, at least in their practices and behaviors if not in theory, to yield to their patients' demands.

Food or diet on which "the *prana* rests" is a central concern. Rarely would an Indian patient not ask his or her physician for a diet, matched to the disease, to go along with medicinal preparations. Almost every pill has to be accompanied by a compatible fluid (like water, milk, or honey) used to swallow the pill. The compounding of mixtures, a lost art elsewhere, is an essential skill of a general practitioner in India because medicine in fluid form is more acceptable to most Indian patients.

The health and illness language of Hindu patients is remarkably Ayurvedic. Hot and cold, light and heavy, dry and wet are the idioms of diets, diseases, drugs, and temperamental dispositions. The Ayurvedic physician is bound by the same medical paradigm from which patients' idioms have emerged. Occasionally, however, a few step out of the fold. A sign in one Ayurvedic physician's dispensary advises his patients that in cases of children's fever (often from infections) it is permissible to mix injections (meaning antibiotics, usually penicillin) with his treatments. Much to the chagrin of purists, many Ayurvedic doctors (*vaidyas*) resort to allopathic medications, even administering injectable antibiotics. Some Ayurvedic medical colleges teach both Ayurvedic and allopathic medicine.

In much of modern medical practice (for example, in the West), scientific and technological imperatives have caused a dissociation of medical practice from the faith traditions of patients and doctors. In India, a variety of medical traditions exist, and only a few patients patronize a particular tradition exclusively. Patients go from a practitioner of one tradition to a practitioner of another, sometimes in the treatment of the same disorder. This "picking and choosing" is not only consistent with the Hindu orientation to life; it also protects against too obvious a fracture between a patient's tradition-informed help-seeking behaviors and the health practitioner's ministrations. Of greater concern than a fracture between faith and medicine in India may actually be the degree to which medicine has been captive to the paradigms of the Hindu philosophical and religious ethos. The successful introduction and widespread acceptance of allopathic medicine point to some unmet medical needs and significant gaps in the effectiveness of traditional medicine against a variety of diseases.

The compendia named after Caraka and Sushruta, along with the *Ashtangahridaya* compiled by Vagbhatta, are the principal texts of Ayurveda. These three works, along with three minor treatises and many commentaries and supplements to them, form a large corpus of medical literature spanning almost the entire history of Hindu civilization. Like most other ancient Hindu texts, the *Carakasamhita* and *Sushrutasamhita* are of uncertain date and equally uncertain, but probably multiple, authorship. Scholars generally place them in the first and second century respectively.[7]

We may regard these ancient compendia, like any modern textbook of medicine, as a compilation of the work of many physicians and researchers. We must assume that once the principles of Ayurveda were established over a long period of time—perhaps centuries—observations and inferences piled upon each other. These were assembled, in loose-leaf fashion, by many physicians or schools of physicians in a variety of localities. Revised, redacted, and reformulated, these *samhitas* have survived, some as fragments and some as later works attributed to the original compilers

Some writers in India feel that Hindu medicine must be comparable to Western practice if it is to qualify as a scientific enterprise. They also feel it necessary to establish the existence of particular individuals in history and their almost singlehanded creation of medical knowledge. The idea of such knowledge arising out of the mind of one seer amounts to belief in revelation and intuition as the basis of scientific discovery. Attempts to push the dates of these compilations as far into antiquity as possible display an attitude present in most discussions on the origins of ancient Hindu texts.[8] Equally powerful is the impulse to construct mythologies surrounding people mentioned in various texts. These endeavors are also marked by a propensity to establish the priority of Hindu civilization over that of other ancient civilizations in various branches of science.[9]

"The object [of Ayurveda] is to protect the health of the healthy and to alleviate the disorders of the diseased."[10] For Ayurvedic medicine, which held disease to be a manifestation of internal imbalance (due to disruptions of, for example, diet or sleep) and external dependence (on seasons, times, places), the ultimate cure was prevention.

Hindu medicine repeatedly stresses the common origin of humanity and the universe. The human relationship with the environment is intrinsic. The elements that compose the universe also constitute the human body, and hence the laws that govern the elements govern the human world. The five elements, or *bhutas*, having been created and therefore being subject to dissolution, are also a source of misery. In health and illness, the qualities of these constituents are the same inside and outside the body, and the interaction between the two may explain disease as well as cure.

When the *Carakasamhita* asserts that the person is equal to the universe,[11] it lays the foundation for a body construction that flows from the earlier Upanishadic attempts to understand the dilemma inherent in decay and death. Concerning this intrinsic relationship between self and environment, anthropologist Charles Leslie observes that the "great-tradition medicine conceived human anatomy and physiology to be intimately bound to the physical systems. The arrangement and balance of elements in the human body were microcosmic versions of their arrangement in society at large and throughout the universe."[12]

The principles of transformation of the body's material constituents and the continuity of the cosmic elements into the human body were firmly established in Hindu thought at the time of the composition of the first medical compendia. *Space* gives rise to the faculty of hearing, carries the spoken word, is the collectivity of all parts. *Wind* becomes the tactile sensory organ; it is responsible for all movements of the body, and lightness is its property. *Fire* is associated with the sense of sight, the eyes, and the form. It gives rise to emotion and lustre, alacrity and bravery, and is the principle of digesting (or cooking) food. *Water* is associated with taste; it is heavy and cool. It is the source of fluids in the body, including semen, and has the property of being viscous. *Earth,* the fifth element of the body, is linked to smell and has the property of hardness and heaviness.[13] The elements also acquire physiological and psychological properties. The ancient physicians had freely and necessarily borrowed from prevailing philosophical models of the person and the universe.

Later Hindu thought, belief, and practice were profoundly influenced by Ayurvedic formulations. So deep and lasting has been the impact of medical theory that not only are contemporary health-related ideas and behaviors continuous with Ayurvedic constructions but so is the social and psychological life of the modern Hindu. The Ayurvedic model may be the best tool to understand traditional life.

Borrowing from the *samkhya* school of philosophy, reality is divided into an external, undecaying, conscious *purusha,* the essence or spirit, and a created and thus decay-prone, multiform materiality, *prakriti.* Ayurveda completes the material person by introducing a force of consciousness that unites *purusha* and *prakriti.* It is this variable that makes the difference between ordinary materiality and the conscious materiality of the human person.

What is the object of the medical enterprise? Obviously the human body, the "epitome of nature," and its nature must be studied. While asserting the primacy of the cause of consciousness, *purusha,* the Self, the *Carakasamhita* goes on to say:

> Inspiration and Expiration, blinking of the eyes, biological functions, movements of the psyche, the ability to shift attention from one sense organ to another, impulses, concentration, moving to another land in dreams, sound sleep . . . , seeing with left eye and perceiving with the right, desire, aversion, happiness, misery, effort, consciousness, control, intelligence, memory, and I-ness, are the signs of the Self. As these signs are found only in living beings and not in dead ones, the sages have called them as the signs of the Self. After its departure, the body is converted into a lifeless, vacant house. . . .[14]

A clear distinction between the characteristics of life and the characterization of a propertyless or unmanifest Self is lost. We find here an echo of

Upanishadic attempts to define the self as *prana*, the breath as the vital force characterizing life. In the *Sushrutasamhita*, the authors are more explicit. They contend that although the *samkhya* school of philosophy with its opposition between spirit and matter is one way of looking at reality, medical science must give credence to the other systems of explanation.

The Svabhava school asserts that the properties manifest in substances are inherent to them, and no other explanations are needed. This materialist vision proposes that consciousness is a characteristic of matter when organized in a particular fashion. The Ishwarvada school contends that the earth, mountains, trees, animals, hell, and heaven are the construction of Ishwara or God. God, therefore, is the cause of all that is the universe. The Kala school, followed by astrologers and others, claims time as the prime mover; it contends that the beginning, condition, and end of the universe are results of the workings of time. Others believe in accidental causality—that it is not possible to determine the origin and cause of all substances. Still another school proposes that fate is determined by good and evil acts.

Each of these formulations attempts to explain the final cause of the phenomena we observe; all rival the *samkhya* thought which regards the unmanifest as the final result. Among these schools, Ayurveda had to uphold its own position, which was to regard the human body as a manifestation of the five elements. Only on that basis could proper diagnosis proceed.[15] By the time of *Ashtangahridaya* this controversy appears to be resolved, and there is no discussion on the distinction between consciousness and reality.

The quandary of the ancient physician is natural and understandable. No physician can remain unimpressed by the mystery of life. At the same time, practical resolution such as that of Sushruta shows wisdom. The object of the physician is indeed that self "which has been created by the interaction of the male and female germinal substances. The product of fertilization is a conscious self made up of the five elements and that is what we must treat."[16]

THE SUBSTANCE OF THE SELF

The argument that anything other than a material conception of the human person is extrinsic to medicine is spurious, disregards genuine dilemmas, and diminishes attempts to construct a more easily comprehensible reality. The early Hindu physicians were giants who wrestled problems that still perplex us. They avoided simplistic solutions yet proceeded with the task at hand. In doing so the early physicians were at the point of intersection between medicine and metaphysics.

The Hindu person may be visualized as a container of consciousness, a vessel, or a receptacle: the word *patra* means both a person and a vessel. It also means a character in a drama, for the Hindu theory of drama sees an actor pouring himself into a role as into a vessel, becoming that part.

The prime fluid substance is *rasa*. This word, too, has many meanings, including dramatic appreciation. The etymology of the word is offered in the *Sushrutasamhita* as deriving from the root *ras*, meaning to move.[17] In this sense *rasa* is the primary product of digestion of food, and the first product that goes through further transformation. Some scholars have chosen to translate *rasa* as "organic sap": ancient physicians spoke of *rasa* as "the basic substance of the organism."[18] Elsewhere *rasa* means taste.[19] In poetry *rasa* means pathos, sentiment, or emotion. Audiences enjoy a drama by tasting its *rasa*, its mood or sweetness.

As an organic sap and the primary product of digestion, *rasa* moves throughout the body and is found in all body parts—the *doshas* (humors), body elements, waste products, and body reservoirs. It nourishes, satiates, and forms the body. In an attempt to describe functional anatomy, *rasa* becomes blood because of the redness it receives on entering the liver and the spleen.[20] In a further series of transformations, *rasa* becomes flesh, fat, bone, marrow, and finally semen. These seven are collectively called *dhatus*, from the verb *dhru*, to hold, for they hold the body together. In an echo of Upanishadic thought, the body is thus a product of *anna*, food, and is involved in a continuous process of transformations. In introducing a Gujarati translation of the minor treatise *Bhavaprakasha*, one scholar notes that nothing besides food and drink enters the body, and thus these are the most important cause of diseases as well as cures.[21] Food and drink ultimately are converted to that which is nutritive and that which is a waste product. The balance and location of the *doshas*, or humors, as we have already seen, govern the dynamics of health and illness. Ayurvedic physicians lay great stress on regulation of excretion and insist that these impulses not be repressed. *Rasa* and *doshas* move about in the body through channels, distributing nutritive substances and regulating physiological functions. The alimentary canal is a model for all the channels. The body ends up being an input-output system. Food, drink, words, deeds, and thoughts are part of an elaborate exchange between the human and the nonhuman.

The *Carakasamhita* establishes the basic facts and principles of Ayurvedic medicine. The text asserts that the mind *(sattva)*, the self *(atman)*, and the body *(sharira)* are the tripod on which the living world rests.[22] It then enumerates the physical properties of the substances that constitute the living world: heavy and light, cold and hot, unctuous and dry, dull and sharp, stable and mobile, soft and hard, clear and slimy, smooth and rough, subtle and gross, and dense and liquid.[23] Paired opposites, the physical properties assume a continuum of degrees from one opposite to the other.[24] Thus innumerable permutations can characterize any one substance. Other properties are sensory (smell, taste, touch), psychological (wish, pleasure, pain, effort), interactional (distance, nearness, combination, number), and ethical (goodness, activity, and inertia).

These properties led the ancient physicians to visualize the individuality of each object and simultaneously to propound the principle of balance and harmony. In each substance are properties that can be matched with those of the body. Similarities and dissimilarities are the basis of both the disease and the cure. Maintaining a balance of substances in the body and establishing a harmony between the body and its environment became the major task of those who desired a healthful state for themselves and also of the physician. Shiv Sharma, an Ayurvedic physician and historian, suggests that Ayurveda contains the principles of both allopathy and homeopathy, for it propounds the principle of treatment with both contrary *(allo)* and similar *(homeo)* substances.[25] For Hindus every contact, human or nonhuman, has the potential to alter the balance positively or negatively, with simultaneous and inseparable implications for moral and physical well-being. An implication of the inherence of properties that has not been sufficiently stressed is the notion of uniqueness or individuality. In a universe perpetually in flux yet essentially the same, how is one to distinguish one thing from another? By elaborate ordering of the properties (physical, psychological, ethical, and interactional) it is possible to see in every object a set of unique properties. By the same logic it is possible to construct classes of objects that are more homogeneous and oppose them to other classes that in turn are sufficiently different from each other. Persons, drugs, diets, and so on can be further modified by the forces of time and geography, and an extremely contextual, relativistic universe emerges. Any contact between two items in the cosmos therefore has to be appropriate.

DIAGNOSES AND PROGNOSES

The etiology of disorders follows the logic of concentric orbits. People are subject to the laws that govern the universe because they are made up of the same substances. Ayurveda assumes a genetic predisposition in which one of the *dosha*s is dominant and contact with certain elements in the environment may further aggravate the *dosha* to create a diseased state. All diseases are mediated through the final common pathway of the *dosha*s.

The three *dosha*s—*vata, pitta,* and *kapha*—are seen as extensions of wind, fire (heat), and water (moisture) in the environment. The laws governing each element attribute qualities to the body, and an excess of any one produces symptoms of overactivity of that *dosha*. An excess of *fire* will produce fever, redness, burning, smells, and discoloration; an excess of *wind* will produce paralysis, cramps, fainting, deafness, and joint pains; and the symptoms of aggravated *moisture* are drowsiness, lethargy, swelling, and stiffness. Diseases can occur as a result of aggravation of two *dosha*s, or even all three, and in the latter case the disease is usually incurable. Disorders arising from the imbalance of the *dosha*s are called *nija*, or endogenous. Those arising from external causes are *agantu* (coming from the outside), while mental illnesses are the third type.[26]

Diseases that attack a person, the *agantu*, are a result of stings, bites, parasites, accidents, injuries of war, and possession states, whereas those resulting from mental disturbances are innumerable. Fear, anxiety, greed, falsehood, praise, envy, insult, sorrow, and grief—all may alter inner harmony, aggravate a particular *dosha*, and lead to imbalance. The laws of nature operate here as well. Passion and anger give rise to heat that in turn may aggravate fire, sorrow and grief aggravate moisture, and vanity aggravates wind. Intellectual errors, excessive use of the senses, and the consequences of time are also causes of illness. The *Carakasamhita* stresses natural impulses: health consists not in suppression of bodily urges but in suppression of unwholesome mental impulses.[27]

The *Sushrutasamhita* adds to the classification a category of natural diseases corresponding to what the *Carakasamhita* identifies as the consequences of time. Old age and death are seen as natural conditions, as are congenital disorders.[28]

Diagnosis is based on etiology, prodromal symptoms (forerunners of a disease), manifestations of the disease, pathogenesis (the development of pathology), and response to treatment. A physician is advised to take into account the reliability of the patient as a historian and not be too quick to conclude from gross observation. A patient is to be examined in terms of his constitution, the quality of bodily substances (*dhatus*), physical stature, psychological disposition, appetite, stamina, and age. Most diagnostic categories presented by the authors of Ayurveda are based on symptoms: for example, fever, swelling, fainting, paralysis, and delirium. The classification is further elaborated in terms of anatomy, meaning the involvement of different body parts and the three humors.

Ayurvedic therapeutics consists of procedures and medicaments. Purgation, emeses, unction, sudation, blood-letting, and enemas are the principal procedures, preparing the patient for the administration of beneficial medications. The idea appears to be that first a patient needs to have poisons removed, channels opened up, passages oiled, and body parts loosened. Once the body is thus taken apart it is ready for the substances and techniques that put it back together. Ayurvedic pharmacopeia is extensive, including fruits, bark, leaves, roots, and animal products. There is no prohibition against meat-eating. The flesh of birds, fish, and domestic and wild animals may be prescribed (vegetarian laws, particularly prohibitions against beef, arise much later). The basic principle governing treatment is to prescribe something that fills a deficiency in the patient (for example, meat for a patient who is wasting) and that is contrary to the cause of aggravation (for example, unction for dryness).[29]

The ancient physician attended to the psychological environment of the patient and advocated calming and soothing language, chanting of mantras, prayers, and the wearing of charms and precious stones according to appropriate astrological conjunctions.

The doctor-patient relationship becomes familiar and intimate over time. The family physician is drawn into an intimate orbit, made into a kind of honorary family member. The physician becomes a counselor and advisor, and a mutuality develops in which the doctor-patient relationship goes far beyond the consulting room. On the other hand, the modern dispensary or clinic is located on main streets open to public view, conveying not only easy access but also a form of advertising. Today history-taking and most physical examinations occur while other waiting patients sit nearby; little concern for confidentiality is shown in matters of ordinary physical illness. Discussion or examination relating to sexual problems is an exception. Except for modern "private" hospitals the open wards in public hospitals are no different in this matter. A more detailed examination (not a part of the routine of a general practitioner or an Ayurvedic doctor) occurs in privacy.

In the Ayurvedic worldview the human being is continuous with the environment. Medicinal preparations for internal use therefore pose special problems. A *vaidya* uses natural products, usually vegetable products, whereas an allopathic physician uses "synthetic" preparations regarded as very heavy and hot, difficult to assimilate, and prone to have side effects. They attack not only the diseased parts of the body but also the healthy ones. Surgical medicine, unlike internal medicine, has a rich and ancient tradition in Hindu culture; its body-consciousness, however, is more physiological than anatomical. Prosthetic devices have been part of Hindu medicine and mythology, and organ transplants have been well-received wherever available. The psychological and social implications of the match between the donor and recipient in cases of organ transplant need further investigation.

Physicians in India avoid making dire prognoses. Although patients and families are very concerned about medical outcomes and may consult astrologers, anxiety about the future is not restricted to patients. The business of astrology in India prospers because of anxiety over what the future holds.

The Scottish psychiatrist Morris Carstairs, who lived and practiced in India for several years, has discussed what prognoses mean to villagers. Known to be a physician, he was called on to attend a woman "possessed by the devil and in great pain." Carstairs found that the woman was soon to deliver "a very healthy little devil" and so declared. He realized later that his pronouncement that the woman would be all right and that the baby would be healthy had a powerful influence on the villagers. They took his authority as that of "a supernatural power, which is the real agent of cure."[30]

On another occasion he was asked to see a young man who had been ill for some time, diagnosed as having cancer. Carstairs freely gave his prognosis on request. A friend present told him later, "Our custom here is that even if a man is sure to die, we never say so. We always say something like 'If it is God's will, he will get better.'" Carstairs realized then that "just as in the past I had been given credit for a decisive intervention simply because I had uttered a hopeful prognosis, now the reverse was the case. I had committed a serious impropriety in stating that the patient would not recover."[31]

THE STATUS OF THE AYURVEDIC PHYSICIAN

In spite of the yearning for good health and disease-free life ("the cause of virtue"), physicians were regarded with mixed feelings from the earliest of times. While the physicians of the gods, the Ashwins, were extolled for their miraculous powers to heal, to restore youth and vigor, to devise prosthetics, and to cure childlessness, their human counterparts were avoided and maligned. One scholar, Debiprasad Chattopadhyaya, has suggested that the status of physicians was lowered because of their emphasis on the material world, as opposed to the priestly domain of the religious and supernatural. According to Chattopadhyaya, the ancient physician saw the body as an extension of the materials of the universe, obeying the same laws, going through transformations, and adapting to the environment as a way of maintaining equilibrium. Such a materialist pursuit was intolerable for the brahminical orthodoxy, and so the physician became an object of disgust. Chattopadhyaya cites the *dharmashastra* literature, in which the impurity of a physician is submitted as a reason for shunning him, and particularly for rejecting any food offered by him. Their state of impurity was due to physicians' "democratic practice of mingling with the common people." Text after text confirms the priestly hostility toward physicians because their "practice entails promiscuous, unaristocratic mingling with men."[32]

We may extend this argument by asserting that the greatest casualty of the taboos against pollution brought about by indiscriminate "mingling with the common folk" was palpation as a method of medical investigation. In most medical texts palpation is not abandoned, but the data obtained from the physical contact between patient and physician becomes thinner and later almost nonexistent. The bias exists from the times of Caraka, who says, "One desiring to know the remaining span of life of a patient mainly by touch should palpate the entire body with his normal (right) hand or *should get it palpated by somebody else.*"[33] Caraka offers no rationale for the substitution, and even if allowance is made for contagion, this is a remarkable admission on the part of scientists. Taboos against touching and ideas of ritual impurity almost completely outlawed palpation as a method of observation, and intuition and inference were enlarged to proportions greater than what we may expect from materialists.

Physician, drugs, attendant, and the patient form a quarter that can cure a disease.[34] The *Carakasamhita* then elaborates on the qualities of each. A physician must be endowed with "excellence in theoretical knowledge, extensive practical experience, dexterity and observance of the rules of cleanliness." Drugs have to be abundant, effective, and of appropriate composition. An attendant heeds the rules of nursing: manual dexterity, loyalty, and again the rules of cleanliness. Finally the patient must be endowed with good memory, must be able to follow directions, and should shed fear and provide all relevant information. Once the hope of cure has been located in this quartet, the text rushes to place the physician at the center of the drama: the physician is like the potter making a pot, a process in which clay and wheel also figure.[35]

The texts repeatedly emphasize the qualities of a physician, who must be not only knowledgeable in scriptures and experienced in medical theory and practice but also friendly, compassionate, virtuous, and of "high lineage."[36] Devotion to learning and rationality are paramount, and the physician must always be ready to act. The *Carakasamhita* regards the profession as suitable to the three upper castes: brahmins (for the welfare of all living beings), *kshatriyas* (for their own protection), and *vaishyas* (as a livelihood). The *Sushrutasamhita*, on the other hand, also allows *shudras*, the lowest caste, to be physicians. In modern India a physician may be from any caste.

If the virtues of physicians are stressed, the dangers presented by quacks are also often repeated. Talking too much, half-knowledge, pretense, and arrogance characterize quacks, and the texts describe the fate of a patient in such hands as worse than death. Because even the best drug is reduced to a poison when administered badly, "the wise person desiring (long) life and health should not take any medicine administered by an irrational physician (quack)."[37] The Ayurvedic texts spare no words railing against the charlatan. He is a sinner, "wicked and death himself," his medicine is worse than Indra's thunderbolt or the poison of a snake. The *Carakasamhita* states that it is better to immolate oneself than to be treated by an ignorant physician.[38] He kills not only those who are about to die but also those whose time has not yet come. It is hard to say whether the dread of quacks comes from the exclusiveness of a guild or from an attempt to weed out the incompetent to reduce the ambivalence experienced toward physicians.

Like their forebears the Vedic philosopher-poets, the learned physician-authors of Ayurveda were intensely concerned with matter, words, properties, actions, and consequences. Rival schools of thought and a regulated exchange between them appear to have been the order of the times. These considerations attest to the strong intellectual life of the itinerant practitioner. The physician is admonished to "devote himself constantly and without negligence" because "there is no end of Ayurveda."[39] Winning a point and defeating an opponent are also important motivations for the Ayurvedic writers.[40]

The physician's education follows the model of a young man living in the house of an experienced teacher. Advice to the student is precise. He must select the best available treatise and a teacher who can best teach that text. It is important to choose an experienced and knowledgeable physician who is free from censure, conceit, envy, and anger, and who is paternal toward students. The teacher looks for a disciple worthy of being taught. A student should be calm, friendly, "with good-looking eyes, mouth and nasal ridge" (an apparent description of the invading Aryans), without physical defects; devoid of haughtiness, anger, addictions, greed, and idleness; intelligent, dextrous, and sincere, with good reasoning and memory.[41]

The student is instructed in the practice of medicine and principles of conduct. He is to avoid women who belong to others, never to enter the house of a patient without the presence of a person known to the family, to maintain confidentiality, and never to mention a patient's approaching death.[42]

MODERN INDIAN HEALERS

A contemporary Ayurvedic practitioner—almost always a male—does not like his patients to give him too many details of their symptoms. The patient is more impressed when a diagnosis is made with as little information as possible. The actual physical examination consists of inspecting the face and tongue and taking the radial pulse. From his reading of the pulse, a *vaidya* may even tell what the patient had to eat the previous night. The patient at this point is truly impressed by the powers of the physician. A patient's manner, dress, name (which may convey caste, religion, and region of origin), and initial presentation combine with the data from pulse examination to yield a diagnosis of disturbance in the balance of humors.

An Indian *vaidya* I visited recently declared his discomfort with orthodox interpretation of the ancient texts. For him, the current revival of Ayurvedic principles in newspapers and college curricula was no more than unthinking reproduction of the ancient texts with undue stress on the alimentary canal. He provided a set of simple propositions: (1) The human body can possess diseases; (2) The physician must make an effort to cure them; (3) Nature provides the means. Concepts of diseases do change with time, he said, but there are no new sufferings nor has human nature changed. Ayurveda, to him, has become "an old bottle which has been sealed permanently. A patient must desire to be cured and the physician must desire to cure the patient. Beyond that there are no eternal truths. The medical *parampara* (tradition) must be challenged." He added that there was only one eternal truth, that "time was ever-flowing."

This *vaidya* saw every ailment as psychosomatic. Changes in appetite, "heaviness in abdomen," problems of sleep, coughing, joint pains, and headaches were the complaints of his clientele. He had no problem with patients of his taking medications prescribed by another doctor (for example, an allopathic physician), especially for fevers, but he warned them to avoid self-medication. He gave permission for his patients to wear charms and amulets, and "God willing" they will get better. He told his patients, "The cure also depends on your fate, but when you do get better I will get the credit." In his office was prominently displayed his system of classification of diseases and their etiologies, in English. (No etiology is given for worms because the *vaidya* does not consider worms to be caused by a psychological imbalance; they are the only condition caused by external factors.)

Diseases	Reasons
1. Piles, fissure, fistula	Having doubts and allegations about seasons, circumstances, food and medicines
2. Dysentery, amoebiasis, colitis	Impatience, longing for perfection and precision beyond necessity, sticking to ideals and principles beyond necessity and limits
3. Hysteria, epilepsy	Negative thinking, self-abuse, nagging

4. Skin disorders   Wrong thoughts (dirty thinking)
5. Diabetes   Ego
6. Troubles with joints   Deep interest in psychology, philosophy,
                             astrology, and medical science
7. Breathing troubles   Self-medication
8. Worms

After examining his patients he prescribed for them. I did not find that he was burdened by the principle of "informed consent." His patients were compliant and grateful, though he regularly prescribed diets considered contraindicated in popular beliefs (for example, buttermilk in cases of asthma). Patients understood that they must not argue with him or talk back to him.

Relaxing after the day's routine, he spoke freely. He was a very popular *vaidya* and had a thriving practice. His father and grandfather were both *vaidyas*. Their education was traditional, the son learning from the father, though he had attended an Ayurvedic college and left without graduating. He invited me to sit in on his father's clinic if I wanted to observe a more traditional practice, quotations from the texts, and the mixing of astrology with medicine. [43]

The Ayurvedic texts decried the scourge of quackery, but this *vaidya* found self-medication to be the greatest problem. The popularization of Ayurveda in a host of publications and vernacular newspapers (which devote a full page to Ayurveda at least once a week) has given the people handy home remedies for a variety of conditions. This popularization, coupled with the unregulated dispensing of Ayurvedic medicines and the principle that naturally occurring substances and ordinary dietary items have in them the potential for health and illness, has made informal exchanges of recipes and regimens the norm. I was not surprised by this physician's concern about self-medication. It is usually easy to obtain allopathic drugs from pharmacists, who sometimes are asked by patients to suggest medications. There are instances in which physicians' "compounders" (assistants who compound medication and attend to dressing wounds) or pharmacists have opened their own roadside dispensaries. I remember one such compounder who hung a shingle that declared "just like a doctor." For patients with everyday illnesses, over-the-counter drugs and a man with "some experience" is good enough. The more like them he is, the easier he is to approach. The specialists, allopathic consultants, are approached with fear and trepidation, though the consulting rooms of a good many of them are crowded. The maverick *vaidya* is not easy to approach, but then his formal manner of seeing each patient privately (unlike the custom of his father and other general practitioners who hold a sort of court) gives him a mystique and power.

The example of this *vaidya* is instructive because he represents the more recent transformations and adaptations in Ayurvedic practice. He is unorthodox in his challenge of existing dogmas, but his attempts to incorporate new experience are part of the intermingling of traditions so common in India.

Many physicians, including my medical school contemporaries practicing in India, have shared with me their impatience with very talkative patients. To them the patients appear very anxious and "most of them need somebody like you [a psychiatrist]." The patient's intolerance for pain and uncertainty about outcome drives him or her to elaborate symptoms endlessly. If patients are impressed by a physician's ability to divine a diagnosis with minimal information, so are they put off by his reluctance to listen to their preoccupations. On one occasion a surgeon returned from abroad asked the wife of a patient to stop "putting on an act" as she was tearfully explaining her worries about her husband's health. Later the surgeon cynically explained to me that he knew the "drama" was to persuade him to reduce surgery fees.

Another common feature of health delivery in India is persons who have achieved the status of healers because of special talents. Their practice is more continuous with modern medicine, but the powers attributed to them are more consistent with folklore. They are specialists in the sense that bonesetters and snakebite healers are specialists: they cater to a particular ailment or disability. Unlike healers who heal exclusively through religious incantations or talismans and the like, their claim to fame is grounded in a more physical and worldly regimen of treatment. In a southern city I found one such example in a retired military sergeant who attracted thousands of men, women, and children suffering from a variety of muscular diseases. At the age of fourteen he was discovered by a guru to have extraordinary powers of healing. The guru himself had such powers and trained the young man in the art of healing fractured bones and muscular diseases by applying splints and unguents to the limbs of injured animals. On one occasion during his service in the British army he massaged a British officer back to health, and his powers became known. On retirement from the army he was provided with quarters to continue the practice of his divine gift.

Among his patients were victims of polio in advanced stages of contractures. Some had birth injuries, some cerebral palsy, and others were victims of malfused fracture and muscular atrophy. In long lines people waited outside the small room where he treated them one by one. Many had camped out in the city and came daily to finish the course of treatment. He massaged their deformed muscles and joints using a sanctified ointment. He hardly ever spoke aloud when ministering to his patients but usually muttered something. He later told me that he repeated a secret *mantra* at each treatment. Often he broke contracture (the rigid shortening resulting from scar tissue formation) with a jerk, and the scream of the patient was taken as an indication of closeness to cure by the people outside.

At an open playground nearby he had an elaborate and ingeniously contrived physiotherapy set-up. After being massaged by the healer (called "doctor" by his patients), the patients and their families walked or were carried to the playground for their exercises. Later he exhorted each patient to try harder and often pricked the diseased part with a pin. He told me he was testing for sensation in the limb.

His language was Ayurvedic. He spoke about the humors, about hot and cold. He prescribed a diet for each of his patients—asking them to avoid sour foods like milk and rice (a staple in South India); encouraging hot foods like meat, fish, eggs, ghee; and expressly prohibiting injections. He combined the divine grace of his guru, his military comportment, the principles of physiotherapy, Ayurveda, and some ideas about muscular diseases from modern medicine.

All patients were treated free of charge. That gave him greater power because he performed the service without personal gain; the transaction was not canceled out by an exchange. He simply gave of himself, his art, and his divine gift. As faith heals fractured souls and spiritless muscles, the general rule in India is that the power of healers is inversely proportional to the fees they charge.[44] Often patients are encouraged to make donations to the cause, but the healer is not to use the money for personal benefit.

What the religious healers take from the patients is their disease, as gurus are often believed physically to take on the diseases of their disciples. Erna Hoch, a Swiss psychiatrist, has practiced psychiatry in India for almost thirty years. A patient once asked that he be allowed to stand with his feet on her shoeless feet and that she put her hand on his head. The patient's request was related to his theory about a cure. Hoch wondered if she were an instrument of psychic dialysis, with the patient's diseased substances passing through her body and being returned to his after purification. Together they could digest the disease.

CARING AND CURING

Most caring for the infirm and the aged occurs within the family. Except in the Buddhist tradition, and especially in the monastic order, at no time in

India have institutions developed for the care of the sick like those in the Christian ministry. Laden with the dangers of pollution and damage to social status, service to the common folk never became an aim of the priestly or religious life. Donations and charity to the poor and helpless are an aspect of good conduct, but personal commitment to service has remained outside the domain of Hindu tradition. The success of Christian missionaries in this regard is an ample testimony to the need for institutions for caring.

Orphanages for abandoned children exist in India and more recently a few homes for destitute women rejected by their families. But these institutions are hardly a celebrated cause. Most survive on meager government support and some on charity. People are believed to have deserved their pain, perhaps because of their sins in a previous life. Compassion for physical, mental, or social suffering is absent, unless it is within the close orbit of the extended family. The lawbooks make any number of references to the physically and mentally handicapped whose sight must be avoided in the performance of ritual ceremonies. The act of service has been a lowly task; those high in status are seen as most deserving of service.

Curing is a different matter. Faith is a major ingredient in healing, and the healer is a recipient of devotion. Healing, especially selfless healing, gives power. There is hardly a corner of India without a shrine, temple, or pond for healing, and naturally the presiding priest performs the necessary ritual for healing physical as well as psychological illnesses. Gurus at established *ashrams,* or places of refuge, provide for many the last hope of cure, as we shall see in Chapter 9.

In matters of healing, Hindus are free to choose the form and practice most congenial to them. Allopathic medicine in India has a vast following: there are more than a hundred such medical schools, with over a half-million hospital beds and over 300,000 licensed medical practitioners. Close to a hundred Ayurvedic colleges exist, with the number of its practitioners slightly below 300,000. Thus their positions are almost parallel (except in the number of hospital beds—about 20,000 for Ayurveda). Most allopathic practitioners, however, are in cities and towns, while the Ayurvedic practitioners are mainly in the rural areas of India.[45] The countless other healers at the periphery of both medicine and religion—the bone-setters, snakebite healers, spiritual masters, *mantrikas* (those who use *mantras* to cure or remove a spell), and exorcists—complete the health delivery system in India in the smaller villages.[46]

But there is a more important point of departure. From the perspective of the consumer, allopathic medicine is good for acute conditions and Ayurveda for chronic conditions.[47] The overwhelming preference for allopathic physicians and medicine in acute conditions, especially those that appear to be life-threatening, is a result of that medicine's effectiveness in controlling infections, fevers, bleeding, and the problems of difficult childbirth. Conversely, conditions become chronic only when they fail to respond to treatment. Not only are multiple theories invoked to explain them, but multiple treatments also prevail. A system of medicine that addresses internal states of disequilibrium as a consequence of the totality of life (food, sleep, diet, states of mind, relationships, stars, *karma*) more closely corresponds to the indigenous system of explanations.

·8·

Karma, Death, and Madness

Whence are we born? Whereby do we live, and whither do we go?
Svetasvatara Upanishad

DEATH AND DYING

If the ethical problems concerning the issues at birth are confounding, those at the other end of life are relatively simple from a Hindu perspective. Not that death does not produce bewilderment and anxieties in the dying and sorrow and loss in the surviving, but the religion long ago found a way of coping with death by denial of its finality. In the Hindu consciousness, death is not the opposite of life—it is the opposite of birth. The two events simply mark a passage.

In time everyone must go—when the body is worn out and when one has paid one's accumulated debts to the gods, sages, and forefathers. What *is* seriously mourned is an untimely death. The dead person's age, sex, marital status, and place in the hierarchy, the suddenness of death, and the quality of life help to determine responses to the death. Helplessness produced by death or impending death is coped with after the fact by the thought of an eternal *atman* or rebirth.

Not long ago I was grieving over a personal loss and had occasion to observe these two distinct but related attitudes. Letters and telegrams from far-flung relatives made a special note of the undecaying character of the *atman*, the self of the deceased, and included quotations from the *Gita:* "The self is not killed when the body is killed," and "Those who are born have to die and those who die will be born."

A seven-year-old granddaughter of the deceased remained somewhat unaffected for the first few days. When the clan gathered as part of the mourning ritual, however, the young girl suddenly realized the implications. She asked her mother tearfully, "Why are these people here?" The mother, who was the daughter of the deceased, responded with tears, and then she knew. She began sobbing and screaming, asking for her grandfather in a heartrending way. For the next few days she was somewhat withdrawn, but she carried on her person a drawing she had made of her grandfather and asked questions both at home and at school about the fate of those who die. "What is *atman?*" she asked, and "What is rebirth?" A week or so later her grief was resolved. She came home from school one day and announced to the entire family that her grandfather would soon be reborn. She said that one of her cousins or aunts would soon be pregnant with a male baby and that he would be her grandfather. In a flash I realized that in her childlike simplicity she had captured the age-old Hindu idea of rebirth—that death was denied.

In the Hindu ethos death is a concern not only for the dying but also for those close to the dying. Those who attend the seriously ill are very conscious of this dimension and carefully conceal or reveal the facts about the patient's condition. The family's and the physician's task is to nurture the will to live. The will may be sapped by a physician's declaration of helplessness. A physician usually asks the family to call to the bedside "all those who need to be present." The impending death is not explicitly pronounced because words have power. Naming death may invite it too quickly.

It is difficult to imagine a controversy either between ethicist and physician or between family and physician on an issue like "Do not resuscitate" orders. (It is true that modern technology has not yet arrived in India for mass consumption and that it exists only in the rare hospital being equipped for the practice of a physician returning from the United States. But this alone does not explain the absence of controversy.) The Hindu is generally allowed to die peacefully, for artificially or mechanically sustained life is held to be of little value. Most people prefer to die in their own beds. (A few very wealthy Indians may make "air-dashes" to the United States for transplants and bypasses, or a young man with wife and children may, when stricken by a fatal illness, invite heroic efforts if the family can afford it at all.)

Ayurvedic texts are unequivocal in advising physicians to abandon all treatment when symptoms of approaching death appear. Their reasoning is uncomplicated. Diseases are classified as curable and incurable. With the latter the physician is advised not to waste effort and resources. This advice is not without self-interest, for "the physician treating an incurable disease certainly suffers from the loss of wealth, learning and reputation and from censure and unpopularity."[1] A terminal patient should not be given medication, but if the relatives of a dying patient insist, the physician may allow some nutrition to sustain the body.[2] If it appears that a patient is near death, the physician is advised not to respond even to a messenger coming to fetch him.

THE WORKINGS OF *KARMA* AND THE ROLE OF THE *GUNAS*

Inexplicable illnesses and untimely death, like accidents and misfortune, are explained by the unseen workings of *karma*. *Karma* is a theory of causality. The moral consequences of past action leave residues that influence future events. Whether now or later, all actions must be paid for, and it is assumed that unforeseen events are due to deeds in a previous life. The *Carakasamhita* accepts the theory of rebirth on the grounds that perception is limited, while the scope of the imperceptible is large and can only be known by scriptures, inference, and reasoning.[3]

In the medical texts, action springs from three main desires: desire for self-preservation, desire for acquiring means for a comfortable life, and desire for a happy state in future existence.[4] The attainment of these aims depends on right conduct. Attention is focused on the realities of this life, for *daiva* (the fruits of action from a previous life) can be mitigated by human efforts. The rules of righteous conduct involve an obvious emphasis on medical principles: adequate and nutritive diet, exercises and activity, rest and sleep, moderation in sexual conduct, and avoidance of excessive greed, anger, and sorrow. As philosopher of religion Surendranath Dasgupta suggests: "Right conduct is not conduct in accordance with the injunctions of the Vedas or conduct which leads ultimately to the cessation of all desires, or through right knowledge and extinction of false knowledge, but is that which leads to the fulfillment of the three ultimate desires. The cause of sin is not transgression of the injunctions of the scriptures, but errors of right judgment or of right thinking."[5]

A more difficult problem for the authors of the Ayurvedic texts was untimely death. Was it to be explained by *karma?* A strict adherence to the theory of *karma* would decree a predetermined time of death for everyone. Then the efforts of the physician would have no meaning, but neither would prayers and good conduct. Here the authors come down squarely on the side of effort and free will, the result depending on a combination of the nature of *karma* and the effectiveness of treatment. In an interesting twist of argument, the ancient writers reinforce the idea of good conduct, in accord with the models of virtuous men and the wise and moderate use of the senses. Neither the gods nor the spirits of the nether world inflict disease on a "person himself unaffected by his own deeds." A person should be regarded as the cause of his or her own intellectual errors and hence "the doer of happiness and unhappiness."[6]

People in India do not passively wait for their *karma* to manifest itself. *Karma* is more often invoked as an explanation after the fact; the failure or incurable illness is explained by unseen *karma.* Both elite and common folk pursue personal happiness and work to avoid pain. They may resort to means consistent with their beliefs and therefore appear fatalistic to some, but they do try to eradicate disease.

A notable exception to this interpretation of *karma* is the explanation of epidemics. Epidemics result from the collective misdeeds of a whole community; they are lapses of *dharma* (social order) on a mass scale. The kings and priests who serve as models for the masses are held particularly responsible for leading the people to violations of *dharma.* This after-the-fact explanation is similar to Hindu explanations of unexpected, unusual, or seemingly unrelated events. Those unaffected during an epidemic are said to have accumulated good deeds, thereby securing protection. During an epidemic, people are exhorted to truthfulness, charity, observance of celibacy, and attention to discourses on scriptures as part of an effort to avoid the disease.[7]

The theory of *gunas* (the qualities of goodness, action, and inertia) has a bearing on ethical behavior. Actions are consistently seen as substantial; they accumulate on a person's ledger of deposits and debits. Hindus explain good and evil acts either as errors of intellect or as the result of an innate disposition. In the realm of moral actions, the determinants are *gunas.* The Ayurvedic descriptions of psychological personality types produced by the dominance of a particular *guna* leave little doubt that there are ethical implications.

The collective action of the *gunas* imparts a particular natural disposition in which is a propensity for a certain set of actions. This brings us back to action, for the *gunas* have a feedback mechanism: their manifestations have consequences, and so does action. If the natural law, derived from the *gunas,* unfolded as a process of internal dynamics, there would be no need for a theory of ethics or the laws of *karma.* But several factors intrude upon such a natural dynamic. A person comes into contact with food and with other human beings, and purity and impurity are derived from such contacts. Specific actions have to be undertaken to restore the original equilibrium when contact is made with impure objects. According to Dumont, contact with organic states and substances (birth, death, food, sleep, excreta, corpses, dead animals) brings about temporary impurities for some and permanent impurity for others. Persons in a state of long-term impurity include those whose occupations expose them to constant contact with such substances as leather and animal flesh.[8] Impurity is thus both an attribution according to the values of a society and a result of specific interactions with the environment. The state of impurity in itself is not sinful, and in most instances temporary impurity can be removed by a ritual bath. A hierarchy of values and status is nevertheless in operation. Low-caste people may seek to raise their status by taking on jobs considered to be more pure, and impurity may be seen as a form of penance.[9]

The impurity associated with organic states has an intrinsic relationship with two fundamental biological processes, desire and hunger. At the very beginning of creation, we saw that desire was the first seed of creation, the falling apart of Prajapati. The hierarchy of the castes also derived from the relative value of his body parts. Desire, particularly sexual desire, brings about a change in the inner equilibrium of *doshas* and *gunas* and must therefore be remedied.

Hunger was also a motive for creation, for hunger personified death and was averted by eating. Hunger and desire, associated with death and birth, have the greatest potential for altering a person's substantive nature and must be remedied to avoid states of sin.

Finally, the great equalizer time is the cause of all disturbances in the equilibrium of *gunas*. Organic states, birth and death, biological impulses, hunger and desire—all are functions of the passing of time. Not only death, the ultimate tragedy, but the repeated cycles of hunger, desire, and satiety, the tragedies of everyday life are wrought by time. Kali, the mother-goddess of India who takes her name from *kala* (time), is the great destroyer.[10] Time brings about differentiation and dissolution, and standing still does not effectively maintain, let aside enhance, the qualities of *gunas* and the store of *karma*.

In worldly affairs we must constantly strive to avoid the dangers of pollution, and we must battle the ravages of time. Pain and suffering, old age and death are consequences of the workings of biology and time. To avoid states of sin and attain good health, virtuous conduct is essential. Modeling one's self after a religious soul *(dharmatma)* may be an easier answer than following *dharma* which is so prone to change.

THE HEALING OF MADNESS

Unmada is the category of mental illnesses in the Ayurvedic literature.[11] The word suggests its proximity to *mada*, alcohol. The texts describe separately the disease of alcoholic intoxication, but the word *unmada* (excited by *mada*) suggests that the model of mental illness may have been derived from states of acute alcoholic intoxication. The classification of mental illness conforms to the Ayurvedic categories of *nija* (endogenous, arising out of the imbalance of *doshas*) and *agantu* (exogenous, mostly possession states). The conditions that lead to disturbances of *doshas* include unsuitable foods, tantric practices applied improperly, diseases that make a person weak, and states of anger, greed, fear, grief, anxiety, and excitement. Also those who are "frequently injured or whose minds get damaged" are susceptible.[12] This kind of insanity is defined as a "wandering about" of mind, intellect, consciousness, and memory. When the insanity arises from the disturbance of wind, the symptoms include constant and incoherent speech, foaming at the mouth, inappropriate smiling, laughing, dancing, and singing (we may say the person is flighty). Anger, excitement, violence, running about, and a desire for cooling things describe a disturbance of bile, that is, the person is excessively heated up. Standing in one place, mutism, oozing of saliva, minimal movements, and excessive sleep are manifestations of phlegm-induced insanity; the person is in the grip of inertia. Or the patient may have a combination of these symptoms and etiology. Except for the last, these types of insanity are considered curable and are treated with appropriate and corrective dietetic regimen, unction, emesis, massage, enemas, reassurance, and a variety of drugs—the standard Ayurvedic repertoire.

The other type of insanity, caused by the wrath of gods or ancestors, or possession by various categories of spirits, is regarded as incurable. Some say that this insanity is caused by "inauspicious action done in previous life" and also by "intellectual errors."[13] The insanity-inducing agents try to incite the patient into violence, pleasure, or worship. Such patients may be filled with unusual energy, excessive strength, and speech. People become susceptible to possession states because of faulty habits, states of sin, inappropriate performance of rituals, and the touch of impure or inauspicious persons and creatures, and they are especially vulnerable when they deliver a child or when they see family, city, or country destroyed. The treatment includes drugs, recitation of *mantras*, offering to deities, vows, performance of rituals, and worship of gods.

The temple of Chhotanikora is about twenty kilometers inland from the port city of Cochin in the state of Kerala on the west coast of India. Kerala's population is almost 50 percent Christian, including Roman Catholics, Syrian Christians, and Protestants. Cochin is just a short hop south of Calicut, where Vasco da Gama landed in 1497 on his first sea voyage to India "to seek Christians and spices."[14] The most common name among the Christians is Thomas. Legend has it that the apostle of Christ, St. Thomas (the doubting Thomas), came to India. Cochin is also a home for Jews, who claim origins there in the early centuries of the Christian era.

The temple of Chhotanikora is well known in the area as a place of healing for the mad. Situated on a busy street of a small town, the temple is part of a large complex. I was allowed into the temple, in spite of my beard (usually associated with the Muslims, who also form a sizable minority in the state), my American wife, and very American-looking children. I couldn't produce my sacred thread, but the temple priest took my word for it when I said I was a brahmin and could recite the *gayatri mantra*.

Surrounding the main temple are rows of rooms on both sides, the guest rooms where the patient and his or her family live during the treatment. I observed a few patients standing in catatonic postures and some milling around. I could not speak to them because of the language barrier, but a few young enthusiasts eager for conversation with a "foreign type" filled me in on some details.

The insane are brought there and given a room if available, at nominal cost. On the day of the healing ceremony they bathe in a small pool of almost stagnant blackish water and are brought before the healing priest. The priest is in a state of trance, his body swinging and shaking. A patient presents himself or herself to the priest, who divines the cause of madness. The patient also has to get into a trance to communicate with the spirit of the priest, who encourages him or her into a state of "shakes and tongues."

Once the patient is in rhythm with the priest, a dialogue occurs about what has possessed the patient. (My informants told me that they themselves did not believe in "ghosts and spirits.") The standard treatment is for the patient to drive iron nails into the wooden pillars around the site of the ritual, or else into a big banyan (Indian fig) tree, with their bare palms or foreheads, the number of nails depending upon the severity of the case (usually measured by the reluctance of the "spirit" of the possessed to talk with the priest in trance). The patient goes back for a second course of treatment if the first fails to produce a cure.

I asked whether some patients were never cured and received a somewhat hesitant answer: "They don't stay long enough to get a complete cure."

"Nails," I asked, "with bare palms and foreheads?" The young enthusiast showed me the tree and the pillars, and on them was hardly any room for new nails.

"Don't they bleed when they hammer the nails like that?" The answer: "Sometimes."

"But why nails?" I received no satisfactory answer to this question either from them or from a psychiatrist living in the United States but originally from that area. The nearest approximation was that possession of an iron object was supposed to keep the ghosts away.

I could not help speculating on the crucifixion, a powerful symbol on a coast that has known Christianity and has had an active church life for centuries. Symbols with power to heal—the crucifixion and the resurrection—may have been blended into the healing ritual of a Hindu temple.

The healing of madness in many places in India is just such a multi-religious mixture. Muslim *pirs* and *babas*, Christian saints, Hindu gurus, ponds and rivers, temples and shrines together form a collage of healers and healing sites. Some healers derive their power from presiding over a ritual at a sacred site; some sites receive their fame from the presence of a renowned healer.

Sudhir Kakar has described in detail the healing rituals at the temple of Balaji in Rajasthan and the everyday work of a Muslim *pir* conducting his clinic in the shadow of a mosque in the old city of Delhi. The temple at Balaji, Kakar tells us, is renowned for its tradition of healing madness. Patients are brought there by their families, who stay nearby in charitable inns. Some are violent, some withdrawn; others speak and gesticulate inappropriately, apparently engaged in conversation with the spirit of the dead person possessing them.

Kakar compares the healing ritual to a judicial proceeding. It begins with an application. The patient offers food, part of which is returned to the patient after it has been brought into contact with the idol of Balaji, the presiding deity. The power of the god is thus transmitted to the patient, facilitating the next stage of the appearance *(peshi)* of the *bhuta*, the possessing spirit. If the spirit does not appear, the patient makes a petition that requires payment of additional sums of money. Thus "the application and the petition rituals incorporate the awesome authority of the gods in their demand that the patient go into a trancelike state of *peshi*."[15]

Once the *bhuta* appears, announced by a violent shaking of the patient's body, a struggle may ensue between the *bhuta* and the god, and the *bhuta* may agree to leave or may stubbornly oppose the power of the god. In the process the assembled community joins in the rituals, provoking and insulting the spirit and praising the deity's power. The next phase in the ritual is the confession or statement, in which the spirit declares the sovereignty of the god and agrees to leave the patient alone.

This healing ritual is a struggle between the all-good and the all-bad. But evil is an intrusion, and the patient only a passive victim. The possessing spirit may be a close relative recently passed away, or a more alien spirit.

From a clinical point of view these patients represent heterogeneous conditions—from conversion disorders to schizophrenia. Those with less serious conditions recover rapidly, others may take time, and in some others a more malignant *bhuta* may later replace the one dispatched successfully. Neither the family nor the community and its priests regard the patient as

evil. Some vulnerability, physical or emotional, or perhaps a special attachment of the departed spirit to the patient explains the state of possession.
The possessed patient is not in a state of sin, only a state of weakness, and this
is often explained by astrological conjunctions or the working of *karma*.

Both folk and classical understandings focus on the unfulfilled states of
those who died premature or accidental deaths. They died without realizing
their ambitions and passions, including hatred and a wish for retribution.
They enter the bodies of those best suited to fulfill the unsated desire or to
thwart the designs of those left behind.

Indian psychiatrists have reported an epidemic of possession in a village
near Ranchi in Bihar. In the most common form, in which a woman feels that
a goddess is coming, she avoids her husband, fasts, sleeps on the floor,
becomes dishevelled, curses or blesses people, and becomes hyperactive.[16]
Other psychiatrists have encountered the syndrome in patients at the All-
India Institute of Medical Sciences in New Delhi. They stress the sudden
onset, the change in the behavior of the patient (she seems almost a different
person), and the possessing spirit who makes various demands of the relatives.[17] Both reports point out that the "faith healer" is the first resort of the
family. A significant feature of the syndrome is the patient's leverage in
bringing the behavior of other family members into compliance with her own
wishes, the least of which is to "get them off her back," as the American
idiom goes.

RELIGIOUS MADNESS

Religious and ecstatic states have often been mistaken for ordinary madness. The distinction is not always clear, as cultures draw the line at different
points. In India there is a tendency to see unusual actions and feats, especially if they involve the defiance of rules of self-interest, as manifestations
of a religious soul. Prolonged fasts, firewalking, lying on a bed of nails,
rejection of sexuality, subjection of the body to prolonged deprivation and
pain, abdication of common status roles—all these are evidence of a liberated
soul. Even in the possession syndrome (either by definition of folk culture or
the Ayurvedic texts) one can be possessed by a god or a goddess. Unless the
associated behaviors are gross, destructive, or violent—in short, unless they
disturb social harmony—one's possession by a deity insures for the person
the role of a diviner, healer, or giver of blessings.

The distinction based on social harmony is important. Those who act
against the family, group, or village, as opposed to the scriptural commands
of *dharma*, are seen as ordinarily mad. The context gives meaning to unusual

behavior and determines the response of the community. It is also important to emphasize coherence and continuity in behavior. Grossly incoherent behavior and speech, and the inability of the "mad" person to display consistently certain behaviors, also become suspect. People later considered saints were not uncommonly taken to faith healers, exorcists, and *vaidyas* during an early period of their lives. The religious leader and mystic Ramakrishna is a classic example. Initially thought insane by members of his family and village, he was sent to both doctors and exorcists. After he began to be considered a saint, his disciples spoke of the religious visions and trances of his childhood as signs of his future greatness.

Historian of religion June McDaniel, in an extensive study of madness and ecstatic states in Bengal, has observed that devotional traditions value certain types of madness as states of ecstatic vision and union with the deity. Among Vaishnavas (those who worship Krishna or his other forms), devotees seek the state of *divyonmada,* divine madness, in which they share the goddess Radha's states of extreme joy and sorrow. Worshippers of Kali seek to share the madness of Shiva and Kali, finding in madness their link to divinity. Bauls, the wandering singers of Bengal, proudly call themselves *ksepas,* lovers of God who have gone mad from religious desire or vision. All these forms of religious madness involve extremes of emotion, trances, and claims of religious identity. Because of the similarity of such states to secular insanity, even saints have been exorcised in their early lives in an attempt to make them seem more normal.[18]

Karma, then, is a system of explanation. Construction of self beyond death was meant to achieve mastery over anxiety about dying, but inasmuch as the body and the ego-self remain, the life-course is subject to disease and dying. Laws of human beings in action need to be formulated in concert with the earlier explanations. In the theory of *karma,* the human spirit once again asserted itself and sought to bring fate within human control. Recognizing cause and effect in everyday action promoted ethical and responsible conduct but also provided a way to link actions from different periods. Furthermore, the theory explained the inexplicable and thereby provided an after-the-fact justification for untoward workings of time.

In medical theory, *karma* is understood equivocally. Resigning oneself completely to fate makes the work of a physician meaningless but leaves many questions unanswered. Therefore only a few medical conditions and epidemics are seen as a result of fate, and human effort is thought capable of overcoming consequences of disease.[19]

Hindus want cures for their illnesses, but they are not satisfied by methods that involve little hardship; a more difficult pilgrimage is able to bring greater good. An injection of penicillin strikes awe, but a difficult dietetic regimen creates respect for the dispenser and begets an accumulation of good actions. The body and mind that are loosely put together are prone to change, always fragile, and subject to the consequences of unknown previous acts; this understanding leads Hindus to define illness as misarticulation. Such bodies and minds have to be broken apart in order to be in correct conjunction and then rebuilt. Fasting, austerities, and penance aid in the process of breaking down the body and mind, purifying them for rearticulation, and adding to a store of good actions. In the healing of madness, *karma* is often invoked as an explanation because the causes of that illness seem less proximal. The Ayurvedic as well as religious therapeutics for the cure of madness bring together these various dimensions.

·9·

Gurus as Healers

What I want to achieve—what I have been striving and pining to achieve these thirty years is self-realization, to see God face to face, to attain moksha [liberation].

Mahatma Gandhi, *An Autobiography*

For Hindus no relationship is marked by as much veneration and significance for well-being as the one between guru and disciple. Every child learns to regard the teacher as the beneficent giver of knowledge and thus a rightful claimant of adoration. Prayers sing the guru's praises. The Hindu trinity—Brahma, Vishnu, and Shiva—are gurus, but the guru before one's eyes is greater than they. Ordinarily understood, the guru is one who teaches, and learning *(vidya)* is ultimately self-knowledge. The guru leads the disciple to the realization of truth, the devotee to the feet of God. Guru Nanak, founder of the Sikh faith (which began in the late 1500s, mainly in Punjab, as both an accommodation of Islam and Hinduism and a departure from some of their practices), declared that in coming face-to-face with the guru and God together, it is the guru that should be paid obeisance first, for through the grace of the guru God is discovered. Gurus are godlike. The state of darkness before the light is like an illness, a state lacking inner cohesion, and the guru is a dispeller of darkness. Therefore a guru is a healer, and thousands flock to him to obtain cures for their maladies.

The power to heal has always inspired awe. A patient in pain, in dread of some disease or inner turmoil, looks to the healer to render him or her whole. Patients, like penitents, attribute power over themselves to those who take away pains, wash away sins, and clear a path to well-being. This tendency to experience the guide, leader, or healer as a repository of special knowledge and charisma is common in the Hindu world. The same might be said of those who care for and cure diseases of the mind—from the tribal healer or the shaman to the psychotherapist.

104

The word *guru* has many meanings. Literally it means "heavy": the *guru* is heavy with knowledge. *Guru* means that which comes first, that which is of primary importance; it means a teacher, a guide, a spiritual master. The Hindu guru bestows knowledge, a state of health, inner cohesion, and goodness.

Many Upanishadic dialogues, as we saw, used the vehicle of a relationship between teacher and apprentice to show the path to self-realization. Transactions between the intellectual and spiritual leader and the student-seeker are intensely psychological and are meant to be equivalent and intertwined. As has been suggested, the guru-disciple relationship is a therapeutic paradigm.[1] We shall approach a fuller appreciation of the role of the guru as healer and teacher through an examination of the *Bhagavad Gita,* the celestial song of the Lord.

HEALTH AS ACTION IN THE *BHAGAVAD GITA*

The *Gita's* dialogue between the warrior-prince Arjuna and his mentor Lord Krishna may easily be regarded as the principal model of the guru-disciple relationship. The transformation from a state of sadness and doubt to a state of conviction and action is the center of the plot. The dialogue is paradigmatic of the Hindu vision of healing through a transmission of values essential to the observance of religious obligations.

Through the centuries since its compilation the *Gita* has often been treated as the epitome of Hindu scripture. Coming at the end of the classical era (around 100 B.C.E. to 100 C.E.), it is considered by many philosophers to be an Upanishad and part of the *shruti,* or revealed literature. Although among the Hindu scriptures there is no single book that parallels the place of the Bible in the Christian tradition, the *Gita* comes closest. It has become infinitely more popular than the earlier Vedic scriptures. Its preeminence in the Hindu world and its drama of psychological healing and restoration through a guru-disciple relationship make it an ideal object of our study.

The *Gita* comes to us as a dialogue between Arjuna and Krishna, an *avatar,* or incarnation of God, who took on human form to deliver the world from decay and danger. The interaction of the two showed how values are transmitted; it erased the doubts of a mortal and energized him to action with the experience of awe and wonder at God's magnificence. Doubt was replaced by certitude. The dialogue is not only a paradigm of how values are transmitted from the guru to the disciple but also an example of how a mythological dialogue permeates the psychology of generations.

The eighteen chapters of the *Gita* are a small fraction of the epic *Mahabharata*, probably the longest poem in world literature, which derives its name from a famous war of ancient times. We hear this dialogue secondhand, as it was related to the blind king Dhritarashtra. The dialogue describes the opening scene of the battle, but actually the *Gita* is set in the epic at a point when the battle was well under way and after Bhishma, the hero of the Kuru lineage, had fallen.

What follows has come to be regarded as the Hindu search for self-realization. Various paths to an understanding of reality, and an adaptation to it, are suggested. The messages of the *Gita* are polyvalent, bringing together many views formerly seen as conflicting (such as *dharma* and liberation, and the paths of wisdom and compassion).

In the *Mahabharata* text, the *Gita* is placed after the death of the elder and leader of the family, and in the middle of a war, when conditions of fragmentation had been well established. In the *Gita*, Krishna proclaims himself the savior of a people disconnected from their moral obligations. The antagonist in the war, Duryodhana, translates the conditions of the times succinctly when he says that he knows what *dharma* is but can't engage himself to perform it, and knows what *adharma* (the prefix *a* meaning "not") is but cannot disengage from it. The archvillain of this epic could not have articulated man's distractedness with more poignancy.

As the battalions of the two armies are assembled, the warrior Arjuna observes men eager for battle. Among those arrayed against him are his relatives, teacher, and elders. He is overcome by great compassion and sadness at the prospect of battling and killing those he loves. His limbs begin to falter and his mouth becomes dry. He puts his arms down and refuses to fight. Krishna then begins a series of arguments to persuade him to take arms, first by pointing to his unmanliness and "vulgar weakness of heart." Afflicted with despair, not knowing the *dharma*, Arjuna asks for guidance: "Pray tell me for sure, pray guide me, your student who asks for your help."[2]

Krishna urges Arjuna to fight on the grounds that when a person is slain, the *atman* is unharmed, because "swords do not cut him, fire does not burn him, water does not wet him, wind does not parch him."[3] When Arjuna remains unmoved by the promise of an understanding of metaphysical reality, Krishna reverts to a more human tactic to persuade the reluctant warrior. In an attempt to shame him Krishna argues that Arjuna will invite dishonor to his name: even death is not worse than ill fame for one who has lived an honored life. But still Arjuna is not shaken from doubt and inaction.

According to the *Gita*, the worldly hero is wise. He has no attachments; for him pleasure and pain, gain and loss, victory and defeat are alike. Exhorted not to care for acquisition and preservation, he has a resolute understanding of his obligations. He does not seek the fruits of his actions. Krishna advocates yoga for the wise hero, to draw away his mind from the objects of sense perception. Yoga, in integrating all the faculties of the psyche through concentration, holds a tight rein over the vagaries of the mind and the ego.

While Krishna's discourse on Hindu philosophy continues, the reluctant and uncertain prince is troubled by what he perceives as a contradition in the message. He has just heard an exposition of a self untouched by worldly events, a self that has come to be ultimately interior and indestructible. But he is also being urged to go to war.

The philosophy fails to energize Arjuna into action. The conversion of the recently acquired knowledge into action bewilders him. How is it his duty to take arms against his elders, teachers, and relatives? "If you hold that insight is superior to action, Janardana [Krishna], why then do you urge me on to fearful action? With quite contradictory words you seem to confuse my own insight. Therefore tell me definitively which is the course by which I will attain to the supreme good."[4]

In the words of Krishna, a perpetual doubter perishes. Krishna proclaims himself to be an actor as well as the creator and maintainer of the universe. Without Krishna's actions the world would be thrown into confusion. Action divested of desire is the principle he propounds.[5] The ordinary consciousness of the actor should be split from his actions. The path of action that does not arise from the dictates of the flesh is deemed superior to the path of knowledge. None can remain free of action, especially those of Arjuna's warrior caste. For attainment of the highest good, work must be done as duty, without desire or attachment. Extolling the heroic virtues and deeds of Arjuna's forefathers, Krishna resorts to yet another worldly motivation for action: to set a model for others to follow. "People do whatever the superior man does: People follow what he sets up as the standard."[6]

Krishna exhorts Arjuna to be full of faith and free of doubt. But the refractory prince does not stop objecting, even when the "supreme secret" of yoga is divulged to him. In the verses that follow, a theory of the *avatara*, the reincarnation of God, is articulated. From age to age, when there is violation of *dharma*, God takes on a human form for the protection of the good and destruction of the wicked. Surrender to God's will, a path superior to those of both knowledge and action, now takes center stage in the dialogue. Doubters and quibblers can be saved only by unquestioning faith. Concentration, meditation, penance, knowledge, sacrifice, and renunciation give way to detached action and to devotion. Knowledge and experience of God can erase all doubt. As Krishna says:

> I am the beginning, the middle, the end, of all beings,
> of words the one syllable
> I am everlasting time
> the wisdom of the self among all wisdom
> of the gamblers I am the dicing game
> of the splendid the splendor
> I am the victory, the resolution,
> the taciturnity of the mysteries,
> I am whatever is the seed of all creatures.[7]

Refuge in and worship of an almighty and incarnate god is a new avenue for the attainment of the highest good. In return for devotion, Krishna resides in the devotee, and the devotee in him. At this point, a change in Arjuna's attitude is suggested. The doubter, no longer reluctant, takes delight in Krishna's words. To become devoted to Krishna is to be a part of him. Arjuna mellows but is not convinced; he is eager for a more personal engagement. Though his bewilderment is gone, he feels an urge to experience the divine. Krishna gives in to the yearning of his pupil and bestows on Arjuna divine eyesight. He then unfolds his universal, endless, mysterious, and tremendous form, dazzling Arjuna,[8] who then surrenders to the Lord's command: "I see you, so rare to behold . . . Immeasurably burning like sun or the fire . . . The person eternal I hold you to be. Obeisance to you, have mercy good God! I seek to encompass you who are primeval." Krishna responds to this surrender with an invitation to the pupil to go on to war: "Therefore arise yourself now and reap rich fame, rule the plentiful realm by defeating your foes."[9] Arjuna asks forgiveness for his rashness, saying he wishes to think of Krishna as a companion; he pleads to be treated as a father would his son, as a lover his beloved.

Returning to human form, Krishna describes the virtues of *bhakti*, worship and devotion, asserting that the worship of a personal god is better than all other paths. Calmed and gratified, Arjuna is ready to accept the values of the earlier message: detachment from worldly desire, withdrawal of senses from the object-world, action without expectation, stable-mindedness, knowledge of the self *(atman)*, and a virtuous life. Arjuna accepts the teaching and is healed. His sorrow and bewilderment vanish, and energized to action, he goes on to war and ultimate victory.

If the *Gita* did not attempt to overturn the established brahminical order, it did open up a new path to gaining energy and certitude in facing suffering and achieving comfort and calmness in face of misery. *Bhakti*, the devotion to a personal god, emerged as an alternative to the early Vedic religion and came to be a dominant trend in the Hindu pluralistic tradition.

The path of *bhakti* allows the common person to share with the community. One scholar suggests that *bhakti* means "to share in, participate in." From the root *bhaj,* meaning "to divide or apportion, to share in," as a *bhakta* shares in his god, *bhajan* is a devotional song and Bhagavan is God himself. The word gradually came to mean sharing with or participating in something or someone with affection.[10] The actual practice of *bhakti* humanizes the god, and as Arjuna asked to be treated like a lover, a union with God as beloved is visualized. A display of affection, at times in torrents and frenzy, characterizes groups immersed in their devotion. Devotional songs *(bhajans)* are daily practices in Hindu households and regularly in the larger community. The theme of merger predominates.

The dynamic between a confused man seeking direction and his chosen guru reveals to us some essential features of healing and action. From a theological perspective, the transformation of a sad and dejected warrior into a victorious hero is an outcome of a personal engagement between the god and his appointed agent. *Nara* (man) and *narayana* (god) are united in a common cause to uplift the languishing moral order *(dharma)* and also save the individual. The inevitable erosion of order in the world is the work of time.

Krishna declares himself to be an *avatara* (appearance) who comes to deliver the world from the chaos generated by entropy.[11] As with mortal beings, time takes its toll on institutions, affirming their proneness to decay. The Hindu idea of cyclical ages implies repeating and deteriorating time-spans and, in the spirit of the *Gita,* requires a savior who destroys evil and protects the good. The person in the scheme of the *Gita* is an agent without an independent will, an instrument of divine design. It would seem that only a few are chosen to carry out the will of God at a time of crisis.

A deeper understanding of the *Gita* dialogue reveals to us the utter helplessness of human beings. Even those who seem to oppose the will of God are also part of an intricate design to resurrect and renew the cosmic order.[12] If the powers of the supreme are displayed in a terrible splendor, so are the relentless and inevitable effects of time. God is also time beyond death, as Krishna says. Creation and destruction are but a phase in eternal time.

At the social level the *Gita* presents a conflict between spontaneous action arising out of emotional and social attachments and action arising out of ancestral obligations. The quandary is resolved in favor of duty to maintain social order, to counteract time. Disorder comes from swimming against the current. A hierarchical society is legitimized.

At the human and personal level the *Gita* points to the dangers of attachments and to the need for selfless action. Knowledge and action have been redefined, and Vedic thought gives way to devotion to a personal god. If the *Gita* gives sanction to a caste society, it also provides for the lower and the lowest strata of the social order a way to self-worth and self-esteem via union with a god. Self-surrender and not doubt is the way to approbation.

THE SEARCH FOR A GUIDE

Our understanding of the Hindu person is also enlarged by the rich tradition of *bhakti* in later Hinduism.[13] The self is defined here in terms of relationality. In Indian devotional religion two aspects of the self are emphasized. There is a deeper or "true" self, which is seen in relation to a deity, and a more superficial and conditioned self based on social transactions. Both god and guru represent this deeper self, and a merger with the god or guru is also a merger with the deeper self.

Among goddess-worshippers the person's religious self is based on relationship with the Mother. The mother-goddess is worshipped in many forms, as a young girl or as a powerful mother. The devotee is a favored child always on her lap, pouting yet loving. Among worshippers of Shiva, the person may be a devotee and servant of the god or a beloved, or the person may merge with Shiva in blissful union.

For Vaishnavas, there are several possible roles. The devotee's religious self may be a loyal servant of a great lord, a parent of a divine child, a friend of a friendly god, or a lover of a beloved. Realized in meditation, this self comes to be the true self, especially for renouncers. The more ordinary sense of ego, the phenomenal self, is a tool used for social interaction.

The worldly or phenomenal self is associated with *kama*, lust toward worldly persons and things. It is for persons trapped by the world of illusion (*samsara*) who have not yet recognized their spiritual depths. The true self is associated with *prema*, unselfish or spiritual love, in which the person seeks detachment from worldly objects and directs all love toward the deity.

The goal of *bhakti* self-transformation is dissolution of the bodily self and its rebirth as an agent of the spiritual self. This self exists in relation to the deity and participates eternally in mythic events. Because it may be realized during life, death becomes unimportant, something that affects the false self but cannot touch the true one. After the *bhakti* transformation the false is not really false—it has become a servant of God.

The devotees in the foregoing discussion themselves become gurus over the course of time. Theirs is a full-time occupation to seek union with their particular deity. In the *bhakti* tradition the *Gita's* mandate of conduct according to dharma is set aside, while seeking oneness with God becomes paramount. If not quite anticaste, the *bhakti* movement downplays those distinctions in favor of personal engagement with a preferred object of idealization. In this manner, the gurus of the various traditions become otherworldly. They try to reach the far shore of the stream of life, negating involvement in ordinary pursuits and thereby establishing a selfless orientation to life, a prerequisite for admiration and adoration. Their actions on this side of the shore often go against tenets of good conduct (for example, their sexual mores), implying a deliberate affront to the ethics of *dharma*.

The devotees grounded in *samsara*, the common folk, seek a union with their chosen gurus. Irrespective of their own caste status, their spiritual pursuit gives meaning to their lives, lifting their (usually) lower status and esteem. *Gurupat*—that which falls from the guru or the energy transmitted by the guru—has the potential for transforming and healing the devotee.

The search for a guide in India is intense and almost universal. Not only those who have renounced the world but also elders, teachers, and leaders are idealized. It is necessary for such persons to demonstrate selflessness, for even from a distance and without a face-to-face engagement devotees will surrender themselves to their exemplars. Mahatma Gandhi was for many in India just that sort of person. His vows of celibacy, his donning a loincloth, and his renunciation of private property established his selflessness. He too searched for a guru, someone he could enthrone in his heart. According to Gandhi, the guru commands the entire being of a pupil: there can be no doubting, no questioning, only surrender. Then the pupil is molded into the image of the guru. A favorite devotional hymn of the Mahatma was a song written by a medieval Gujarati poet-saint, Narsimha Mehta. In this hymn truthfulness, nonpossession, compassion, sexual restraint, and stable-mindedness are the virtues of a true devotee. Gandhi made these the prerequisites of leadership. A guru has to overcome self-love and pride and be concerned with the welfare of those who trust the guru with self-abandon.

In the hierarchy of encounters, the *Gita* asserted the primacy of affective experience. Such an experience made for a communion from which commitment arose. Knowledge and understanding as the sources of detached action became meaningful later. The primacy of the affective experience in the development of Hindu thought and psychosocial life marked a crucial departure from the foundation of religious pursuits established before the period of the *Gita*. It cannot be overemphasized that any social, ideological, or theological change in India never quite completely displaced the earlier tradition. But a new path to "attaining the highest good" did become established as a dominant mode of worship. The ideas of the *atman* and *ahamkara* as two selves were also reinforced by the *Gita* and continue to shape the psychosocial contours of Hindu life.

·10·

Epilogue: Being Together and Being Well

I must have been about seven years old when my parents decided to perform the thread ceremony for my older brother. I was old enough to receive the sacred thread but my horoscope, according to the family astrologer, suggested that I was not ready: the moon was not in the correct conjunction, "did not reach high enough."

Other transitions fill my memory. My older brother, in the final year of high school, planned to go to the university. Living in a dormitory would have been too alien, so the whole family moved from a village to the city. Summer holidays assumed special significance as the time we returned to our village, the ancestral home where I had grown up. During that first summer at home the thread ceremony for my brother was performed. The first sacred occasion under my father's leadership of the family (after his father's death) meant great fanfare, including the return of other families of our caste and many relatives.

One evening several of my cousins and I were playing a variation of "cops and robbers" on the sandy riverbed. One player became unusually enthusiastic and accidentally hurled a stone that hit me on the side of the bridge of my nose, missing an eye by a fraction. I was hurt and bleeding. My playmates panicked and urged me to prepare a version of events to meet the barrage of questions we would encounter on returning home. The impending ceremony must have been what prompted me to ask a slightly older playmate, who already had his "thread," to press down on the wound and recite in his mind the *gayatri mantra*. Mystery surrounded this *mantra*, which the father whispered into the ear of the son receiving the sacred thread. It was never uttered aloud; it was a divine gift, a mark of one's brahminhood. I thought then that the *mantra* had mysterious powers of healing that could stop my bleeding.

Recently, on hearing of an illness of mine four decades later (separated by seven oceans, as she says), my concerned mother wrote to me. She inquired

113

about my well-being, but more important, she prayed for it. On the top of the letter were inscribed the verses of the *gayatri mantra*.

This was a surprise to me. Women were not supposed to have received the *mantra*. Only the men of the higher castes, the twice-born, received this sacred gift. I later learned that things in India have changed. A resurgent Hinduism favored the recitation of the *mantra* by women. And my childhood fantasy that the *mantra* had healing power was not original or fantastic. The chanting of the *mantra* has been regarded as medicinal, though the style of chanting has changed from private to public and audible. Recently a relative informed me of a modernist explanation. The chanting of the *mantra* stimulated the pineal gland (corresponding to the third eye of the god Shiva, who it is said had obtained immortality by totally awakening the gland). For ordinary people, the stimulation of pineal secretion enabled them to combat disease and lengthen the life span. I did not realize in my childhood that this *mantra* was an important part of sacred Indian lore, a part of the most revered *Rig Veda*.

Religion and medicine in India have been inextricably intertwined. Prayers are not simply a way of obtaining divine grace or the blessings of a deity, for the words themselves have power. They create an alteration in the space that carries them, a change in the mind and body of those who recite and hear them. The Vedic Hindus performed sacrifices to enhance and control the cosmic order, which included physical well-being. Sacred charms and blessed talismans were worn around the neck or arm to ward off diseases and drive away evil influences.

Hindu ideas about health and illness spring from the construction of the Hindu universe. Unlike Western notions of religion, Hinduism is not primarily about the relationship of human beings with a divinity. The religion accounts for the relationships among all that is contained in the universe and the universe itself. Without a book, a prophet, or "a well-knit religious order embodied in a church or in a distinctive class of priests and scholars enjoying divine authority as the ultimate arbiters deciding issues of spiritual validation or social praxis,"[1] Hinduism has survived as a continuous tradition because of its understanding of relationality.

To be together is to be well. In life, where the anxiety of falling apart always looms large, to be well is to be whole as a self—body and mind, inside and outside; to be together in the corporate life of the family, which is also a body; and to be in continuity as a family with the tradition of the lineage. Cohesion and coherence are opposed to fragility and fragmentation. The Hindu tradition over its long history has stressed the ideals of cohesion and connectedness to counter the natural devolution of things and people into parts. Entropy and fragmentation were the way of all flesh. The person and the family had to strive to hold themselves together. Soon after India became an independent country, there was a cry for national integration to hold together the diverse parts of the nation, the society, the polity, the traditions.

But the business of well-being is a full-time occupation. Physical health can easily be disturbed by the wrong kind of food, a change in habits, or disturbed sleep although strict adherence to the order of input and output can usually maintain a state of balance. The social world is also in a state of constant flux: "going with the flow" is not a passive activity. The universe of family and caste is so finely knit and rules are so clearly defined for almost every situation that only in the private world can a person be totally free. The task of seeking spiritual well-being in India is therefore a very private affair. As McKim Marriott observed after his time in a village in North India, "Extreme stability of caste and kinship leaves individuals fairly free to think and to believe as they please. Thus, within one family there may be devotees of as many different gods as there are members; one member of the family may know nothing and care nothing about the god worshipped by another member."[2] Sometimes, I might add, there are *more* gods worshipped within a family than there are members.

Within the stream of Hindu life lie the subjective realities of Hindu persons. Where Ayurveda and *dharma*, along with other constructions of the cosmos, govern the aims of Hindu life, a fluid interpersonal world emerges. This contrasts with the solid world of modern Westerners in which stability, consistency, definite boundaries, and the ability to maintain one's shape or identity are the qualities of persons or individuals. Hindu persons are "dividuals": they easily combine with other people and things.[3]

Human activities and relationships are a grid of intricate hierarchies and boundaries, not always fixed. Such a grid may be visualized as a template for well-being.

The body is viewed as a vertical axis in which the head and foot are the two poles. Head is high, foot is low, higher is purer and more subtle, lower is impure and gross. Who the head of a family is, to whom the headship passes, what one may or may not touch with the feet, to whom and when one bows the head, and at whose feet one sits—all these are connected with the maintenance of well-being.

Instead of the ego-boundaries of an individual, Hindus erect social and geographic boundaries. Prescriptions for the egress of impulse seek to regulate otherwise volatile substances. Limitations are placed on sexual and social intercourse in order to create conditions of social and physical well-being. Crossing these boundaries brings ill health and pollution. Not long ago, a Hindu who crossed the sea was required to go through a purification ritual. On his return from England Mahatma Gandhi faced such a requirement; refusal would have meant outcaste status.[4] Limits, order, and control are essential for human welfare, and trust is founded on the understanding of these boundaries. This is especially true in Hindu society.

Castes and sects represent codes of relationship, as does the family. They give meaning to interpersonal conduct, communal behavior, and spiritual quest. Hindus allow many ways of being religious, yet there is an orthodoxy in the context of a group like a family, sect, or caste. Religion does not enforce absolute laws, either in worship or in relationship. Hindu gods do not demand an absolute adherence to particular modes of being. It is the social consideration of belonging to a group that tends to codify behavior. Medical beliefs and native cures constitute the forces that provide continuity between the past and the present. They cut across geographic as well as group boundaries, for they grow out of a common and enduring heritage of notions about context and relationality. Hindus would readily agree that their medical concerns are rooted in their common religious beliefs.

In closing we may reflect on some problems that surface. In the modern, transitional society, the old norms of relationships no longer work well. The nature of work has changed, and a democratic polity rests on egalitarian not hierarchical, values. Industrial and urban growth has curtailed group cohesion and discouraged traditional behaviors, aspirations, and expectations. A new ethic has not yet emerged, but in the family, where health is a shared phenomenon and connectedness a prime virtue, there is hope for new norms to grow.

In matters of health and illness the problems facing most Hindus are those of a Third-World developing country—problems of adequate nutrition and basic medical care. India, with vast areas of remote villages, is divided by a lack of easy transportation. Not only is medical care inaccessible, it is far too expensive for the people to afford. If modern and traditional medicines are willing to shed their insistence on purity, as has already happened on the periphery, an affordable, accessible, and effective system of care can emerge. If institutions of caring and healing spring from the popular consciousness of the voluntary sector rather than from a total reliance on government sponsorship, the sense of ownership so achieved will lessen alienation between the institutions and their users. The government's task would then be public health and preventive medicine, and at the minimum, clean drinking water. If not "a chicken in every pot," at least a tap in every kitchen.

A most difficult problem is the lack of legitimization of secular life and institutions. There is a massive distrust of public institutions; for example, the systems dealing with justice, taxes, and city traffic are known for violations rather than for compliance and regulation (court cases are described as coming up in the time of one's grandchildren). When only religious institutions have power and justification, those institutions involved with daily life may be relativized or even ignored. Little emphasis is placed on the justice and dignity of all. Outside the home and family is a no man's land. People of lower castes and outcastes are treated badly, shunned and sometimes beaten, barred from the wells and houses of towns, in spite of constitutional guarantees. Communal madness in India erupts in widespread violence and the conflicts that result from easily reached impasse. With few ways to negotiate and resolve conflicts among competing interests, riots seem to occur without forethought, and masses of people are killed.

Next only to the untouchables, women bear the brunt of problematic beliefs and attitudes shaped by the forces of history. Women are seen as having powerful, uncontrollable urges and lacking self-regulation. Thus the society has constructed roles for them in which they are externally governed, especially in the area of sexuality. They seem to have little control over their bodies and little to say in the choice of marital partner in traditional India. Only when they contribute to generational continuity by giving birth to a male child do they rise in power and status. The problems of women and untouchables are two of India's greatest problems today.

In Hindu psychology, the forces of the Self, the body-self, and the body give shape to spiritual and secular quests. The fear of being alone, without an other to respond, generates hunger for contact. Two separate dramas get played out, one a need for intense intimacy, and another a nagging disbelief in the affective profusion of the moment. The environment never fully satisfies one's need for admiration and idealization. Detachment (*vairagya*) always looms on the horizon as an ideal. Suspicion about the genuineness of responses and the persistent demand for confirmation can display an alienation from the body and from others, which results from the Hindu construction of the self, the mind, and the body. Any physician must take these forces into account when dealing with Indian patients.

The Hindu notion of being religious encompasses at once every aspect of existence and the hereafter. It is possible to be an atheist, to cease to believe in anything divine or sacred, but it is difficult to cease to be a Hindu. Given my bias as a psychiatrist, it would not be an exaggeration to state that Hinduism is a psychology, and that to be a Hindu is to have a particular psychic organization. More than anything else, it is the continuity between doctrines, ideas, and beliefs revealed in their richness and variation in Indian medicine and religion.

Notes

In the notes, short titles have been used after the first reference to a work. Primary sources frequently cited have been identified by the following abbreviations:

AA	*Aitareya-Aranyaka*
Ahr	*Ashtangahridiya*
BAU	*Brihadaranyaka Upanishad*
BP	*Bhavaprakasha*
Car	*Carakasamhita*
ChU	*Chandogya Upanishad*
Gita	*The Bhagavad Gita*
KU	*Katha Upanishad*
Manu	*The Laws of Manu*
Mhb	*The Mahabharata*
RV	*Rig Veda*
Su	*Sushrutasamhita*
TU	*Taittiriya Upanishad*

Chapter 1 / Prologue: A Pilgrimage Begun

1. In spelling out a major distinction between East and West, philosopher William Haas comes closest to appreciating the point of departure: "The western mind fixes the object as the *'objectum'*—that which is thrown against the subject—in a word, the *opposite*. The world surrounding the subject is an objective world. It is independent of the subject. . . . Not so the East's. The East did not so entirely cut the umbilical cord between subject and object. Clearly this means that the East, despite the severance from the magic world, has remained closer to it than the West. To give full precision to this fact it would be preferable in relation to the East not to speak of the object at all. For the term object necessarily implies, with perfect reason in western use, the connotation of the opposite *vis-à-vis* the subject. What corresponds to the object in the West, in the East is better termed—the other. This term indicates that whatever be the distance between the subject and the *other* it can

never turn into the distinct cleavage which separates subject and object in the West."
Destiny of the Mind: East and West (New York: Doubleday, 1956), p. 43.

2. *Valmiki Ramayana*, ed. G. H. Bhatt, 7 vols. (Baroda, India: Oriental Institute, 1960–75), 1.57.60.

Chapter 2 / Historical and Cultural Overview

1. Jawaharlal Nehru, *The Discovery of India* (Delhi: Jawaharlal Nehru Memorial Fund, 1981), p. 59. Diana L. Eck, *Banaras: City of Light* (Princeton: Princeton University Press, 1983), p. 9. Wendy Doniger O'Flaherty employs this powerful image in discussing various approaches to the study of mythology—to decode messages written by "generation after generation." *Women, Androgynes, and Other Mythical Beasts* (Chicago: University of Chicago Press, 1980), p. 4.

2. Nirad Chaudhari, *Hinduism* (New York: Oxford University Press, 1979), p. 63.

3. According to Nehru (*Discovery of India*, p. 74), the word *Hindu* first appears in an Indian book in the eighth century C.E. It occurs in ancient Persian texts much earlier. According to Pandurang Vaman Kane, the word appears in Persian literature around 500–400 B.C.E. (*History of Dharmasastra*, 5 vols. [Poona, India: Bhandankar Oriental Research Institute, 1968–77], 5:1613). I have used Kane's volumes for summaries in this work, often without specific citations.

4. For details on the archaeology of the Indus valley, see Bridget Allchin and Raymond Allchin, *The Rise of Civilization in India and Pakistan* (Cambridge: Cambridge University Press, 1982). Excavations conducted under the leadership of Sir John Marshall from 1924 to 1931 and later in 1946 under the direction of Sir Mortimer Wheeler brought to light the pre-Aryan history of India. Until these discoveries, it was generally thought that the Vedas, the earliest surviving literature of the Hindus, composed c. 1500–1000 B.C.E., provided the most ancient knowledge about India. The excavations showed that the so-called Hindu culture is really a product of the interaction between the cultures of Aryan invaders and the inhabitants of the Indus Valley, an idea still alien to many in India.

5. A. L. Basham, *The Wonder That Was India* (New York: Grove Press, 1959), p. 16.

6. Heinrich Zimmer, *Myths and Symbols in Indian Art and Civilization*, ed. Joseph Campbell (Princeton: Princeton University Press, 1972), p. 95.

7. Ashis Nandy, *Alternative Sciences* (New Delhi: Allied Publishers Private Limited, 1980), pp. 4–5.

8. Suniti Kumar Chatterji, "Linguistic Survey of India: Languages and Script," in *The Cultural Heritage of India*, vol. 1, ed. Chatterji et al. (Calcutta: Ramakrishna Mission, 1958), pp. 53–75.

9. *Brihadaranyaka Upanishad*, trans. F. Max Muller, in *The Upanishads*, Part 2 (New York: Dover, 1962), 6.1.14 (hereafter cited as *BAU*).

10. Fredrick Dunn has used the term *cosmopolitan medicine* for what I have been calling allopathic or Western medicine, and his designation has been adopted by Charles Leslie. See Fredrick Dunn, "Traditional Asian Medicine and Cosmopolitan Medicine as Adaptive Systems," in *Asian Medical Systems*, ed. Charles Leslie, 137–58 (Berkeley and Los Angeles: University of California Press, 1976), and Charles Leslie's Introduction to the same volume, p. 6.

11. Sheryl Daniels, "The Tool-box Approach of the Tamil to the Issues of Moral Responsibility and Human Destiny," in *Karma: An Anthropological Inquiry,* ed. Charles Keyes and E. Valentine Daniel, 27–62 (Berkeley and Los Angeles: University of California Press, 1983).

12. Sarvepalli Radhakrishnan and Charles A. Moore, eds., *A Sourcebook in Indian Philosophy* (Princeton: Princeton University Press, 1957), p. 4.

13. Nehru, *Discovery of India,* p. 79.

14. McKim Marriott, "Little Communities in an Indigenous Civilization," in *Village India: Studies in the Little Community,* ed. McKim Marriott (Chicago: University of Chicago Press, 1969), p. 197.

Chapter 3 / *Samsara:* The Stream of Life

1. The performer of yoga and the *bhakta* pursue goals at the two ends of a spectrum. One seeks a state of withdrawal of the senses, and the other seeks a pouring out of emotions in a state of extreme devotion. Both involve surrender and transcendence of the ordinary rules of life.

2. *The Rig Veda: An Anthology* 10.190, trans. Wendy Doniger O'Flaherty (Harmondsworth: Penguin Classics, 1981), p. 34. Hereafter cited as *RV* (O'Flaherty).

3. *Rig Veda* 1.105.4–6, 15, quoted in Debiprasad Chattopadhyaya, *Science and Society in Ancient India* (Calcutta: Research India Publications, 1977), p. 57.

4. Kane, *History of Dharmasastra* 1:3.

5. *The Laws of Manu,* trans. Georg Buhler (New York: Dover, 1969), 2.6 (hereafter cited as *Manu*).

6. Robert Lingat, *The Classical Law of India,* trans. J. Duncan M. Derrett (Berkeley and Los Angeles: University of California Press, 1973), p. 6.

7. Jan Gonda, "Indian Religions: An Overview," *Encyclopedia of Religion,* ed. Mircea Eliade, vol. 7 (New York: Macmillan, 1987).

8. See, for example, Chaudhari, *Hinduism.*

9. *Manu* 2.224.

10. Sarvepalli Radhakrishnan, *Eastern Religion and Western Thought* (London: Oxford University Press, 1940).

11. *Carakasamhita,* trans. Priyavrat Sharma, 2 vols. (Varanasi, India: Chaukhambha Orientalia, 1981–83), 1.1.15 (hereafter cited as *Car*).

12. *Car* 1.8.17–29.

13. *Car* 1.11.3.4–5.

14. *Manu* 10.1–73.

15. Kane, *History of Dharmasastra* 2:757–800.

16. Louis Dumont, *Homo Hierarchicus* (Chicago: University of Chicago Press, 1980). For a different interpretation of the caste, see McKim Marriott and Ronald Inden, *Encyclopedia Britannica,* 15th ed., s.v. "caste system." See also McKim Marriott and Ronald Inden, "Toward an Ethnosociology of South Asian Caste Systems," in *The New Wind: Changing Identities in South Asia,* ed. Kenneth David, 227–38 (The Hague: Mouton Publishers, 1977).

17. See, for example, Kane, *History of Dharmasastra* 5:1664–83; Ashis Nandy, "An Anti-Secularist Manifesto," *Seminar* 314 (October 1985): 14–24.

18. Ronald Inden and Ralph Nicholas, *Kinship in Bengali Culture* (Chicago:

University of Chicago Press, 1977), p. 37. The *Laws of Manu* (2.27–28) holds that the sacraments performed during pregnancy and birth are intended to remove the taints received from the parents. Later sacraments complete the process of purification so that the study of the Vedas can begin.

19. *BAU* 6.4.21.

20. *BAU* 6.4.24–28.

21. Kane, *History of Dharmasastra* 2:239.

22. Lois Murphy, "Roots of Tolerance and Tensions in Indian Child Development," in *In the Minds of Men*, ed. Gardner Murphy, 46–58 (New York: Basic Books, 1953).

23. See Allan Rolland, "Psychoanalytic Perspective on Personality Development in India," *International Review of Psychoanalysis* 7 (1980): 73–88; B. K. Ramanujam, "The Indian Family in Transition: Changing Roles and Relationships in the Indian Family: Patterns of Change in the Seventies," *Indian Social Institute* (New Delhi) 2, no. 1 (January–March 1972).

24. Allan Rolland (in "Psychoanalytic Perspective") contrasts with surprise the care and cleanliness inside a person's home in an apartment building with the filthiness of the public areas like the stairwells—a virtual "no man's land"—in the city of Bombay. The practice of throwing garbage, not infrequently liquid, from an upper-story window into the street with total indifference to passersby is common.

25. It will be recalled that Mahatma Gandhi at a stage in his life took to wearing only a very short loincloth. This was for him the demonstration of his identification with the poor masses of India. From early times the elite classes of the society wore an upper garment.

26. Kane, *History of Dharmasastra* 2:351.

27. Ibid., p. 412.

28. Ibid., p. 427.

29. In most of southern India these prohibitions have not been in force as far as the maternal side of relations is concerned. A maternal uncle may marry his niece, and first-degree maternal cousins may also marry.

30. Inden and Nicholas, *Kinship*, p. 40. The Bengali proverb: June McDaniel, personal communication with author.

31. Prakash Desai and George Coelho, "Indian Immigrants in America: Some Cultural Aspects of Psychosocial Adaptation," in *The New Ethnics: Asian Indians in the United States*, ed. Paramatma Saran and Edwin Eames (New York: Praeger, 1980), pp. 363–86.

32. *ChU* 8.7.1.

33. Gananath Obeyesekere, "The Rebirth Eschatology and Its Transformation: A Contribution to the Sociology of Early Buddhism," in *Karma and Rebirth in Classical Indian Traditions*, ed. Wendy Doniger O'Flaherty (Berkeley and Los Angeles: University of California Press, 1980).

34. *Kausitaki Upanishad*, trans. F. Max Muller, in *The Upanishads*, Part 1 (New York: Dover, 1962), 1.2. See also Albert Schweitzer, *Indian Thought and Its Development* (Boston: Beacon Press, 1956). In the polymorphous thought of Hinduism there are several variations and elaborations of these ways of the dead, and the foregoing is a generally accepted version disregarding scholastic disputes. For an interesting discussion of these debates, see O'Flaherty, *Karma and Rebirth*.

35. For details of the rite see Kane, *History of Dharmasastra* 4:334–55.

36. David Knipe, "Sapindikarana: The Hindu Rite of Entry into Heaven," in *Religious Encounters with Death: Insights from History and Anthropology of Religions*, ed. F. E. Reynolds and E. H. Waugh (University Park: University of Pennsylvania Press, 1977).

Chapter 4 / The Self

1. *Rig Veda* 10.129, quoted by R. N. Dandekar, "Brahminism," in *Sources of Indian Tradition*, ed. W. T. de Bary et al. (New York: Columbia University Press, 1958), emphasis mine. Hereafter cited as *RV* (Dandekar).

2. The word *brahman* derives from the root *brh*, which means "to grow, to increase, to roar." *Brahman* is that which creates, promotes growth. Heinrich Zimmer suggests that *brmhayati* in classical Hindu medicine denotes the art of increasing the life-strength in weak people, the art of making fat. The doctor fattens *(brmhayati)* those who are thin. Similarly, divinities become *brmhita*, "fattened, swollen, puffed up," by hymns and praises; and men, in return, by blessings. *The Philosophies of India*, ed. Joseph Campbell (Princeton: Princeton University Press, 1969), p. 77.

3. *RV* 10.121 (O'Flaherty), p. 26.

4. *RV* 10.90 (O'Flaherty), p. 29.

5. Joseph Campbell, *Oriental Mythology: The Masks of God* (New York: Viking Press, 1962), pp. 10, 11.

6. See Alfred Collins and Prakash Desai, "Selfhood in Context: Some Indian Solutions," in *The Cultural Transition*, ed. Mary White and Susan Pollak (Boston: Routledge and Kegan Paul, 1986), p. 271.

7. There is uncertainty about the exact meaning of *upanishad*. The use of the two prefixes *up* and *ni* before the verb *sad*, meaning "to sit," gives an idea of sitting *(sad)* down *(ni)* near *(upa)*, or to paraphrase, sitting down at the feet of someone capable of transmitting the sacred knowledge of the Vedas. Furthermore, there is an interesting twist to the study of the Upanishads, especially concerning its transmission to the world outside India. The credit for the translation of the Upanishads from Sanskrit to Persian goes to Dara Shukoh, son of the Mogul emperor Shahjahan. Shahjahan gave India and the world the gift of the Taj Mahal, and his son gave the translation of the Upanishads, which were eventually translated into French and Latin by Anquetil Duperron. Dara Shukoh met a tragic death at the hands of his younger brother, Aurangzeb, in 1659, barely three years after the translations were complete. Dara, as oldest son, would have come to the throne instead of Aurangzeb, and the history of the Hindu-Muslim relationship in the latter part of the seventeenth century would have been written very differently. These translations and Schopenhauer's writings on them also marked the beginning of the Western interest in the so-called mystical writings of the East. Muller, *Upanishads*, Part 1, pp. vii–xii.

8. The Upanishads have generally been regarded as mystical writings. That they mark an inward-looking era is undeniable, but to label this only mystical is not fully accurate. The Upanishads are more than the ideas of the Self, for they expound the nature of the self (lowercase)—a person with body, senses, mind, and relationships. They are intensely psychological works, attending to both the phenomenal and the transcendent worlds.

9. The word *prani*, meaning "a breathing animal," derives from *prana*.

10. *BAU* 6.1.7–13.

11. *Taittiriya Upanishad*, trans. F. Max Muller, in *The Upanishads*, Part 2 (New York: Dover, 1962), 1.3.2 (hereafter cited as *TU*).

12. *TU* 2.2.

13. *BAU* 1.3.1–16.

14. In a modern Indian language (Marathi), a paralyzed part of the body is called one "over which wind has passed." In Ayurveda paralytic illnesses are wind diseases. I am obliged to Professor Giri Deshingkar for bringing this to my notice.

15. *BAU* 1.3.19.

16. *BAU* 1.5.21.

17. *BAU* 3.7.2.

18. *BAU* 1.5.22.

19. *TU* 1.6.1, *BAU* 2.2.3.

20. *Isa Upanisad*, trans. Swami Gambhirananda, with the commentary of Sankaracarya, in *Eight Upanisads*, vol. 1 (Calcutta: Advaita Ashrama, 1977), p. 1.

21. *Chandogya Upanishad*, trans. F. Max Muller, in *The Upanishads*, Part 1 (New York: Dover, 1962), 6.12.1–3 (hereafter cited as *ChU*).

22. *ChU* 4.3.3.

23. *ChU* 6.8.2.

24. That we are concerned here with self-awareness is attested by another passage in the same Upanishad, which states that the body may be blind, but the self sees. The *Brihadaranyaka Upanishad* (2.1.16–18) asks the question more directly: "When a man is asleep, where is his self, his 'knowing' self which returns when a man wakes up?" As in the *Chandogya Upanishad*, the answer is found in an involution of the senses and mind into "the heart." More interesting, dreaming is used to illustrate the idea that the self is free from the body, because the self can move to different places in dreams.

25. *BAU* 4.3.14.

26. *Mandukya Upanisad*, trans. Swami Gambhirananda, in *Eight Upanisads*, vol. 2 (Calcutta: Advaita Ashrama, 1982).

27. *Katha Upanishad*, trans. F. Max Muller, in *The Upanishads*, Part 2 (New York: Dover, 1962), 1.1.10 (hereafter cited as *KU*).

28. *KU* 1.2.19.

29. *BAU* 1.4.1.

30. *BAU* 1.4.1–3.

31. Heinz Kohut calls this narcissistic realization the need for a "mirroring" relationship. *The Search for the Self: Selected Writings of Heinz Kohut, 1950–1978*, ed. Paul H. Ornstein, 2 vols. (New York: International Universities Press, 1978).

32. Collins and Desai, "Selfhood in Context," p. 262.

33. *TU* 2.1.

Chapter 5 / The Body

1. *RV* 1.32 (Dandekar), pp. 13–15.

2. *RV* (Dandekar), p. 9.

3. *RV* (O'Flaherty), pp. 209–18.

4. See Campbell, *Oriental Mythology*, p. 187.
5. *ChU* 1.1.2.
6. *BAU* 6.4.1.
7. *ChU* 1.9.1. and p. 17n.
8. *BAU* 2.3.4.
9. *BAU* 2.5.10; *TU* 1.6.1.
10. *ChU* 7.12.1.
11. O'Flaherty, *Women, Androgynes, and Other Mythical Beasts,* pp. 156–58.
12. *KU* 2.5.11.
13. *ChU* 6.7.
14. Wendy Doniger O'Flaherty, *Hindu Myths* (Harmondsworth: Penguin Books, 1973), p. 241.
15. *RV* 10.71 (O'Flaherty), p. 61.
16. *Shruti* was also understood as that which was heard without its being spoken, but here the speaker is unseen.
17. *ChU* 2.9.3.
18. *Aitareya-Aranyaka*, trans. F. Max Muller, in *The Upanishads*, Part 1 (New York: Dover, 1962), 2.1.2.14–16 (hereafter cited as *AA*).
19. *ChU* 6.5.1–3.
20. *TU* 2.2.
21. *TU* 3.10.1.
22. *ChU* 4.10.3.
23. Surendranath Dasgupta, *A History of Indian Philosophy*, 5 vols. (Delhi: Motilal Banarsidass, 1975), 1:208–11.
24. Troy Organ, *The Hindu Quest for the Perfection of Man* (Athens: Ohio University Press, 1970).
25. *Bhavaprakasha*, Gujarati trans. Girijashankar M. Shastri, 2 vols. (Ahmedabad: Sastu Sahitya Vardhak Karyalaya, 1981), 1.1.35 (hereafter cited as *BP*).
26. Radhakrishnan and Moore, *Indian Philosophy*, p. 426.
27. Dasgupta, *History of Indian Philosophy*, 1:243–45.
28. *Patanjali's Yogasutra*, with the commentary of Vyasa and the gloss of Vachaspati Misra, trans. Rama Prasad (New Delhi: Oriental Reprint, 1982).
29. Mircea Eliade, *Yoga: Immortality and Freedom* (Princeton: Princeton University Press, 1970), p. xx.
30. *TU* 2.2–5.
31. *Hathayogapradipika*, Gujarati trans. Vasudev Mahashankar Joshi (Ahmedabad: Sastu Sahitya Vardhak Karyalaya, 1957). For a more detailed analysis and interpretation see Mircea Eliade, *Patanjali and Yoga* (New York: Schocken Books, 1975), and *Yoga: Immortality and Freedom*.

Chapter 6 / Sexuality

1. *Kamasutra of Vatsayana*, trans. Richard F. Burton (New York: E. P. Dutton, 1964). Among the medieval texts the *Kokashastra*, composed in the twelfth century, is also called the *Ratirahasya*, "the secrets of Rati," spouse of the love-god. (*Kokasastra*, trans. Alex Comfort [New York: Stein and Day, 1965].) The *Ananga*

Ranga, "the way of the love-god," was written in the sixteenth century by the poet Kalyana Malla (*The Ananga Ranga: The Hindu Ritual of Love,* trans. and ed. Tridibnath Ray [New York: Citadel Press, 1964]).

2. *The Mahabharata,* trans. J. A. B. Van Buitenen (Chicago: University of Chicago Press, 1973), 1.7.113.4–5 (hereafter cited as *Mhb*). Kane argues that this passage refers to a legend the king may have heard and that the theory of an original state of promiscuity is no longer acceptable (*History of Dharmasastra* 2:428).

3. *Mhb* 1.7.113.14.

4. *Mhb* 1.7.113.18. With the dawning of the age of the lawbooks, alongside significant social changes after the early centuries of the Christian era, we find altered standards of socially acceptable sexual conduct. We can see this in the period between the *Kamasutra* and later texts on love and sex. O'Flaherty suggests that a shift occurred between the Vedic period and the time of the *puranas.* She finds a change from male to female sexual dominance. (*Women, Androgynes, and Other Mythical Beasts,* pp. 77–129).

5. Edward Dimock and Denise Levertov, *In Praise of Krishna: Poems from the Bengali* (Chicago: University of Chicago Press, 1967), p. xviii. Reflecting the fondness for classification and typing for which Indian thought is well known, the Vaishnavas divide the *madhurya-bhava* songs into two broad categories: *vipralambha,* the lovers in separation, and *sambhoga,* the lovers in union. These categories are not entirely separable, for separation is present in union and union in separation, but the literature tends to focus upon one aspect or the other.

6. *The Ananga Ranga of Kalyana Malla,* trans. F. F. Arbuthnot and Richard Burton (New York: Lancer Books, 1964), pp. 106–7.

7. Veena Das, "Paradigms of Body Symbolism: Analysis of Selected Themes in Hindu Culture," in *Indian Religion,* ed. Richard Burghart and Audrey Cantlie (London: Curzon Press, 1985), pp. 180–207.

8. Morris Carstairs, "*Hinjra* and *Jiryan:* Two Derivatives of Hindu Attitudes to Sexuality," *British Journal of Medical Psychology* 29 (1956): 128–38. Gananath Obeyesekere, "Illness, Culture and Meaning: Some Comments on the Nature of Traditional Medicine," in *Medicine in Chinese Culture,* ed. Arthur Kleinman et al. (Bethesda, Md.: Fogarty International Center, National Institutes of Health, 1975), pp. 253–63.

9. In the *Ramayana,* when Rama and Sita return to their capital (after Sita has been abducted and kept in captivity by Ravana), a washerman and his wife are overheard expressing their disbelief at the possibility that Sita could have been chaste. Earlier Rama had asked Sita to prove her chastity by walking through fire. Even after the successful completion of this ritual she is exiled to the forest.

10. Mahendranatha Gupta, *The Gospel of Sri Ramakrishna,* trans. Swami Nikhilananda (New York: Ramakrishna—Vivekananda Center, 1942), p. 593.

11. *Srimad DeviBhagavata Purana,* trans. Swami Vynananda, Sacred Books of the Hindus Series, vol. 26 (Allahabad: Bhuvanesvari Ashram, n.d.), 3.5.13–15.

12. Sudhir Kakar, *Shamans, Mystics, and Doctors* (New York: Alfred A. Knopf, 1982), pp. 152, 156.

13. June McDaniel, "*Bhava:* Religious Ecstasy and Madness in Bengal" (Ph.D. diss., University of Chicago, 1986).

14. *Car* 4.3.

15. *BP* 1.1.36.
16. *BP* 1.2.314.
17. *BP* 1.2.32–33, and *Ashtangahridiya*, text with Gujarati trans. Vijayshankar Dhanshankar Munshi (Ahmedabad: Sastu Sahitya Vardhak Karyalaya, 1983), 2.1.3 (hereafter cited as *Ahr*).
18. *Sushrutasamhita*, text with Gujarati trans. Shastri Kalidas Govindji (Ahmedabad: Sastu Sahitya Vardhak Karyalaya, 1973), 3.3.13 (hereafter cited as *Su*).
19. *Car* 3.4.
20. Inden and Nicholas, *Kinship*, pp. 51–57.
21. Iravati Karve, "The Indian Social Organization: An Anthropological Study," in *The Cultural Heritage of India*, ed. S. K. De, V. N. Ghoshal, A. D. Pusalkar, and R. C. Hazra, vol. 2 (Calcutta: Ramakrishna Mission, 1962).
22. *Mhb* 1.7.113.20, 25.
23. *Mhb* 1.7.107.
24. Keith A. Berriedale, ed., *The Mythology of All Races*, vol. 6 (New York: Cooper Square, 1964).
25. Ibid.
26. Sripati Chandrashekhar, *Abortion in a Crowded World: The Problem of Abortion with Special Reference to India* (London: Allen and Unwin, 1974), p. 44.
27. Ibid.
28. Ibid., p. 45.
29. Barbara Miller, *The Endangered Sex: Neglect of Female Children in Rural North India* (Ithaca: Cornell University Press, 1981).
30. The Indian state Maharashtra has recently enacted legislation curtailing the easy availability of amniocentesis. The law permits the procedure only for detection of fetal abnormalities and forbids it for sex determination.
31. Damodar D. Kosambi, *Myth and Reality* (Bombay: Popular Prakashan, 1962).
32. *Manu* 9.89–90.
33. In "Sati: A Nineteenth-Century Tale of Women, Violence and Protest," Ashis Nandy has argued that "the epidemic of sati in the late 18th and early 19th century was mainly a product of British colonial intrusion into Indian society." He suggests that although the rite had been prevalent among the upper classes for the previous two thousand years, it was never a standard practice. Only in the late eighteenth century did the rite assume epidemic proportions, especially in Bengal, where "widows were being drugged, tied to the bodies of their dead husbands, and forced down with bamboo sticks on the burning pyres" (p. 14). He suggests that the epidemic had several predisposing factors: (1) the need to control the population of women of child-bearing age, (2) conditions of scarcity in famine-ridden Bengal, (3) the anomie that resulted from the fast pace of modernization which destroyed older social institutions and relationships, (4) the law, especially in Bengal, that permitted widows to inherit their husband's property, and (5) the family's desire to secure social status and assert piety. He also suggests that the woman herself found relief from a life of humiliation and that the Bengali elite attempted to find sanction for *sati* in the scriptures. His analysis focuses on the ambivalence toward women as both the sexual and the maternal, epitomized in the split in the image of the Bengali mother-goddess into a nurturant and a destructive aspect. But the most important for him is the influence of Western culture and power, which eroded traditional values and support,

made Hindu men feel weak and impotent, and assailed the cultural sense of both masculinity and femininity. Ashis Nandy, *At the Edge of Psychology: Essays in Politics and Culture* (Delhi: Oxford University Press, 1980).

Nandy fails to make a convincing case that the British colonial intrusion resulted in the epidemic of *sati*. Apart from the fact that the British (whose methods as historians are different from those of Indians) must have begun recording and dating the incidence of *sati* and that they had different sensibilities from those of the nineteenth-century Bengalis, Nandy himself implicates the Bengali psychological response to the infusion of modernity. For Hindu social phenomena we must look into Hindu psychology. To hold the British intrusion responsible for the Hindu response projects onto them the conflicts inherent in Hindu society.

The more important contribution of this paper is Nandy's demonstration of a connection between the psychological development of Ram Mohan Roy and the origins of his commitment to the eradication of *sati*.

Chapter 7 / Ayurveda: The Hindu Medical Tradition

1. *Su* 1.15.33.
2. *Car* 1.30.22.
3. *Atharvaveda*, trans. Acharya Vaidyanath Shastri, 2 vols. (New Delhi: Sarvadeshik Arya Pratinidhi Sabha, 1984). See also Rajchatra Mishra, *Atharvavedame Sanskritic Tatva* (in Hindi) (Allahabad: Punchnad Publishers, 1968).
4. Moriz Winternitz, *History of Indian Literature*, 3 vols., trans. Subhadra Jha (Delhi: Motilal Banarsidass, 1967), 3:626.
5. *Car* 1.6–17.
6. A hymn to the Ashwins refers to the fact that they had brought mortals back from death, from the ocean, from a fiery pit, and had rejuvenated the sage Cyavana, who had become prematurely old. This mythological reference is still alive in the Ayurvedic medicinal preparation called *cyavana-prash*, said to restore vigor and vitality. The Ashwins are closely associated with Indra and have many similar qualities. In the same spirit of rejuvenation, they restored to an impotent man the capacity to procreate, cured blindness, and built divine prosthetic devices (*RV* (O'Flaherty), 1.116).
7. According to Winternitz, the oldest dated medical texts were found among manuscripts discovered in Central Asia and were written in the second half of the fourth century C.E. (*History of Indian Literature* 3:629). Julius Jolly commented on the findings of Bower (called the Bower manuscripts), suggesting that they were "probably written by traveling Hindus in the Indian Gupta script about 450 A.D., according to paleographic criterion" (*Indian Medicine*, trans. Chintamani Ganesh Kashikar [New Delhi: Munshiram Manoharlal, 1977], p. 18). Among the texts was a treatise on garlic and the preparation of eye lotion and a lengthy text on various medicinal drugs and preparations. To both Winternitz and Jolly the available evidence suggests that the formalization of medical knowledge occurred during the Buddhist era. Similarly, they argue that medical knowledge was evident in earlier religious literature, notably the *Satapatha Brahmana* and the *Atharva Veda*. The evolution of ideas about the body's parts and functions can be traced even to the earlier texts, for speculation about the body and mind must have begun

with the earliest efforts of poets and philosophers to grapple with the problem of their existence and the universe around them.

Winternitz places Caraka in the first century C.E., and the Committee of the National Institute of Sciences of India has accepted this date for the *Carakasamhita* (Priyadaranjan Ray and Harendra Nath Gupta, *Carakasamhita: A Scientific Synopsis* [New Delhi: National Institute of Sciences of India, 1965], p. 3). Scholars in the field generally agree that the oldest known text, available in a later rendition, is attributable to Dridhabala of the ninth century. Concerning the *Sushrutasamhita*, it is assumed that Sushruta was somewhat younger than Caraka and that the text now available to us is based on an eleventh-century redaction.

Vagbhatta, compiler of the *Ashtangahridaya*, is placed in the eighth century, and Madhava, compiler of the minor Ayurvedic treatise *Madhavanidan*, in the ninth century at the latest (Jolly, *Indian Medicine*, p. 9). Winternitz, on the other hand, suggests that there may have been an older Vagbhatta at the beginning of the seventh century and a younger one in the eighth century (*History of Indian Literature* 3:635). He claims this on the basis of two texts, the *Ashtangasangraha* and the *Ashtangahridaya*. Both authors, according to him, were probably Buddhists. He places Madhava in the eighth or ninth century. For the *Sarngadharasamhita*, a date of the thirteenth century is asserted by Jolly, and Winternitz agrees. The minor treatise *Bhavaprakasha* of Bhavamishra is accepted as a sixteenth-century work.

8. Chaudhari, *Hinduism*, pp. 27–41.

9. In preparing this work, I have come face to face with these propensities in Indian translations of ancient texts. I have had to sift through them to understand what the original might have meant, for the translators tend to modernize the ancient concepts with the intent of imputing to the ancient construction what is consistent with modern understanding. The idea of microorganisms is an example. The word *bhuta*, used in the Ayurvedic texts to refer to demonic beings coming to existence from the undelivered *jivatmas* of the dead ("those that have become"), has been construed to mean organisms in Priyavrat Sharma's translation of the *Carakasamhita* (p. 241).

10. *Car* 1.30.26.

11. *Car* 4.4.13.

12. Charles Leslie, ed., Introduction to *Asian Medical Systems* (Berkeley and Los Angeles: University of California Press, 1976), p. 4.

13. *Su* 3.1.16–20.

14. *Car* 4.1.70–74.

15. *Su* 3.1.11.

16. *Su* 3.1.11.

17. *Su* 1.14.9.

18. Chattopadhyaya, *Science and Society*, p. 53. Jean Filliozat also uses the word to mean organic sap. *The Classical Doctrine of Indian Medicine*, trans. Dev Raj Chanana (Delhi: Munshiram Manoharlal, 1964), p. 187.

19. Filliozat, *Classical Doctrine*, p. 27.

20. *Su* 1.14.5.

21. Prabhashankar Nanbhatt Gadhadavala, Introduction to *BP*, p. 10.

22. *Car* 1.1.46.

23. *Car* 1.1.49.

24. *Car* 4.6.10.
25. Pandit Shiv Sharma, ed., *Realms of Ayurveda* (New Delhi: Arnold-Heinemann, 1979), p. 15.
26. *Car* 1.11.45.
27. *Car* 1.11.41, 37.
28. *Su* 1.1.17.
29. *Car* 3.1.13.
30. Morris Carstairs, "Medicine and Faith in Rural Rajasthan," in *Health, Culture and Community*, ed. Benjamin D. Paul (New York: Russell Sage, 1955), p. 112.
31. Ibid., pp. 122–23.
32. Chattopadhyaya, *Science and Society*, pp. 246, 241.
33. *Car* 5.3–4 (emphasis added).
34. *Car* 1.9.3.
35. *Car* 1.9.6–13.
36. *Car* 1.29.7.
37. *Car* 1.1.127.
38. *Car* 1.9.15.
39. *Car* 3.8.14.
40. *Car* 1.11.17.
41. *Car* 3.8.4–8.
42. *Car* 3.8.13.
43. For a similar example of a *vaidya* in action see Mark Nichter's excellent description in "Negotiation of the Illness Experience: Ayurvedic Therapy and the Psychosocial Dimension of Illness," *Culture, Medicine and Psychiatry* 5 (1981): 5–24.
44. McKim Marriott, "Western Medicine in Northern India," in *Health, Culture and Community*, ed. Benjamin D. Paul (New York: Russell Sage, 1955), p. 261.
45. *India 1985*, comp. and ed. Research and Reference Division, Ministry of Information and Broadcasting (Government of India, 1986).
46. Morris Carstairs and Ravi Kapur, *The Great Universe of Kota* (Berkeley and Los Angeles: University of California Press, 1976).
47. Harold Gould, "Modern Medicine and Folk Cognition in Rural India," *Human Organization* 24 (1965): 201–8; Harold Gould, "The Implications of Technological Change for Folk and Scientific Medicine," *American Anthropologist* 59 (1957): 507–16.

Chapter 8 / *Karma*, Death, and Madness

1. *Car* 1.10.8.
2. *Car* 5.9.16.
3. *Car* 1.9.6–7.
4. *Car* 1.11.13.
5. Dasgupta, *History of Indian Philosophy* 2:405.
6. *Car* 2.7.19.
7. *Car* 3.12.20.
8. Dumont, *Homo Hierarchicus*, pp. 46–64.
9. The purity and pollution associated with certain tasks have implications for the

regulation of self-esteem and social status. This was illustrated recently in the state of Punjab, when the chief minister of the state, Surjitsing Barnala, was asked by the heads of the Sikh temple to clean the shoes of the members of the community at the Golden Temple. This was a form of penance for his role in the desecration that occurred when Indian troops marched into the temple to flush out Sikh extremists seeking refuge there.

10. *Su* 1.6.2.

11. *Car* 2.7.4. It is not my intent, nor does the scope of this work permit me, to speculate on the correspondence between ancient Ayurvedic categories of insanity and modern allopathic classifications of disease. Such attempts have been made, but outside the broadest comparisons of areas like psychoses and neuroses, the efforts remain very speculative. For example, see O. Somasundaram, T. Jayaramakrishnan, and M. Sureshkumar, "Psychiatry in the Siddha (Tamil) System of Medicine," *Indian Journal of Psychological Medicine* 9 (1986): 38–45.

12. *Car* 2.7.10.

13. Ibid.

14. Percival Spear, *A History of India* (Harmondsworth: Penguin Books, 1978), 2:19.

15. We may note here that as the earlier form of exorcism incorporated Christian elements, Kakar's example shows the incorporation of Muslim terminology and concepts. Kakar, *Shamans*, p. 66.

16. L. P. Varma, D. K. Srivastava, and R. N. Sahay, "Possession Syndrome," *Indian Journal of Psychiatry* 12 (1970): 49–70.

17. J. S. Teja, B. S. Khanna, and T. B. Subramanyam, "Possession States in Indian Patients," *Indian Journal of Psychiatry* 12 (1970): 70–87.

18. See McDaniel, *"Bhava."*

19. Mitchell Weiss, *"Carakasamhita* on the Doctrine of *Karma,"* in *Karma and Rebirth in Classical Indian Traditions,* ed. Wendy Doniger O'Flaherty, 90–115 (Berkeley and Los Angeles: University of California Press, 1980).

Chapter 9 / Gurus as Healers

1. J. S. Neki, "Guru-Chela Relationship: The Possibility of a Therapeutic Paradigm," *American Journal of Orthopsychiatry* 45 (1973): 273–90.

2. *The Bhagavadgita in the Mahabharata,* trans. J. A. B. Van Buitenen (Chicago: University of Chicago Press, 1981), 24.2.7 (hereafter cited as *Gita*).

3. *Gita* 24.2.23.

4. *Gita* 25.3.1–2. Because it mixes ideals and obligations, the problem of action continues to be troublesome in Hindu ethics. Franklin Edgerton was unpersuaded by the idea of a duty commanded by God because inherent in such a commandment was the acceptance of human inequality. After all, the prince was asked to act in a warriorlike manner simply because he was born to fulfill his given obligations. Edgerton finds the *Gita's* answer to the problem of the grounds for action inadequate; he empathizes with Arjuna's questioning that if the path of understanding were superior, why was he urged to act, especially if the morality of duty leads to war and killings? Edgerton observes: "Why indeed, should one fight and slay even 'unselfishly'? This eminently reasonable question is shamelessly dodged by Krishna; no

real answer is given—perhaps because none can be given." *The Bhagavad Gita,* trans. Franklin Edgerton (New York: Harper and Row, 1964), p. 162.

Raojibhai C. Patel has attempted to answer Edgerton's question. First he acknowledges Edgerton's implicit assertion that neither logic nor reasoning are the basis of action in the *Gita.* He then argues that once the mind is stripped of sense-perception and cognition, turned from inference and reasoning, and asked to disregard feelings of attachment, the only basis for action left is memory—racial memory or that of early childhood experiences. He finds the method adopted by the *Gita* as neither analytical nor empirical, neither observational nor logical. "It is past masquerading as all eternity." Not only is one inspired to act in the manner of one's forebears, but the substances of which a person is made impels one to act in a particular manner. "Personhood in the *Gita,*" paper presented at the Seminar on the Person, University of Chicago, 1978.

5. It has been argued that the path of action without desire was alien to the Hindu tradition existing at the time of the *Gita* (Chaudhari, *Hinduism,* pp. 256–59), but an alternative explanation might be more appropriate—that a rationale developed for the enforcement of an established order: the lawbooks commanded one to perform caste-assigned duties without doubt or personal rancor. Once again the Hindu eye was turned toward its past to curtail hierarchic disequilibrium.

6. *Gita* 25.3.21.

7. *Gita* 32.10.20–39.

8. The "mysterium tremendum" of the revelation of Krishna to Arjuna is regarded by Rudolf Otto as a "blending of appalling frightfulness and most exalted holiness" (p. 62). In discussing this "theophany of terrific grandeur" (p. 186), Otto asserts that Arjuna's request to comprehend God's universal form is not granted. This does not appear to be an accurate reading of the *Gita.* Arjuna's request to behold the grandiose form was granted. A common Hindu yearning to see God "eye-to-eye" derives in part from the example of Arjuna. Other mythologies and folklore describe many instances in which a god or a goddess appears to devotees after years of austerities and penance, usually in a benign form. See Rudolf Otto, *The Idea of the Holy,* trans. John W. Harvey (New York: Oxford University Press, 1958).

9. *Gita* 33.11.16–31, 33.

10. R. C. Zaehner, *The Bhagavad Gita* (London: Oxford University Press, 1969), p. 181.

11. In Gujarati the verb of the same origin as *avatara* is *avataravu,* which means "to be born."

12. Any number of myths from the *puranas* illustrate this paradox. For details see Wendy Doniger O'Flaherty, *The Origins of Evil in Hindu Mythology* (Berkeley and Los Angeles: University of California Press, 1976).

13. McDaniel, *"Bhava."*

Chapter 10 / Epilogue: Being Together and Being Well

1. Dhirubhai L. Sheth, "Hinduism: An Ecology of Existence," Paper prepared for the United Nations University project on the Perceptions of Desirable Societies in Different Religious and Ethical Systems, Tokyo, 1987.

2. Marriott, "Western Medicine in Northern India," p. 248.

3. McKim Marriott, "The Open Hindu Person and Interpersonal Fluidity," typescript.

4. Mohandas Gandhi, *An Autobiography: The Story of My Experiments with Truth* (Boston: Beacon Press, 1957), p. 90.

Glossary

Ahamkara. Literally the utterance of the word *I*. An aspect of the self that corresponds to the phenomenal world, like the psychoanalytic ego.

Allopathy. A term commonly used in India to refer to Western medicine with origins in Greek tradition, so called because contrary drugs are used in treatment as opposed to similars, which are used in homeopathy. It is also called cosmopolitan medicine to avoid an East-West dichotomy.

Artha. One of the four aims of Hindu life: purpose or wealth.

Ayurveda. The Indian system of medicine (literally the knowledge of long life). Not curative medicine only, it emphasizes prevention of disease and maintenance of well-being.

Atman. The transcendental aspect of the self, the inner spirit or soul, the immaterial and undying core of the self, a fragment of God.

Bhakti. Devotional worship. A personal relationship is assumed between devotee and God. The word is derived from *bhaj,* meaning "to divide" and therefore "to participate in."

Brahma. The creator God.

Brahman. The creative principle, often the creator; literally that which expands; the infinite.

Brahmin. The highest of the four castes, traditionally associated with learning, teaching, and the performance of religious rituals.

Dharma. Virtue or duty—one of the four aims of Hindu life and as such the ground for all action, the law; literally that which holds together a person, a family, a society.

Dharmashastra. Collectively the lawbooks or texts on *dharma,* composed, revised, and redacted over centuries, beginning in 300 B.C.E. *The Laws of Manu* is one of the better known collections.

Dosha. In Ayurvedic medicine, a humor. Wind, bile, and phlegm together are called *tridosha;* they govern health and illness by their balance and equilibrium.

Guna. An intrinsic quality residing in all substances. The three are goodness, energy or activity, and sloth or darkness. They are invoked in discussing ethics of behavior and in setting up principles of therapeutics, especially dietetics.

Jati. A subcaste; one of the many divisions, permutations, and proliferations of the original four castes. Many derive from occupations and were later incorporated in the formal order.

Kama. One of the four aims of Hindu life: pleasure, sexual impulse. Kama is the god of sexuality.

Karma. A theory of action that propounds a causal relationship between acts. It occupies a central place in Hindu ethics in this life and beyond.

Kshatriya. The second highest of the four castes: the rulers and warriors. They are the protectors of virtue, order, brahmins, women, and cows.

Moksha. The ultimate of the four aims of Hindu life: release, deliverance, freedom from the cycle of births.

Prakriti. Matter, that which has been made; in the *samkhya* school of philosophy, one of the two principles of the universe, the female principle.

Prana. Literally breath, hence the vital aspect of life, also meaning the essence, the principle of consciousness.

Purusha. The creative principle in *samkhya* philosophy representing consciousness. Creation begins when *purusha* combines with *prakriti* (matter).

Rita. One of the oldest concepts in Hindu thought, from the *Rig Veda*. It is the order inherent in the universe, the rule or basis of human conduct and nature, precursor of the concept of *dharma*.

Samhita. A collection, a compendium. The early Vedic texts are referred to as *samhita*, as are the medical texts.

Samkhya. A dominant ancient Indian school of philosophy, probably indigenous to the people before the arrival of the Aryans and later incorporated into Hindu thought. It proposes two primeval entities: materiality and consciousness. Because it is more materialistic, it was an important source of medical theory.

Samsara. "That which flows well." The word is used for the life course, for the collective family and extended network of relationships and obligations in this world.

Samskara. The rites of passage that prepare and renew a person for subsequent stages of life; there are generally sixteen from conception to cremation.

Shiva. A principal god in the Hindu pantheon, iconically represented by a phallus, hence a creator, but associated also with destruction.

Shraddha. The rite for dead fathers, carried out by a son immediately after the death; it involves feeding, gratifying, and thus embodying the dead. The ceremony usually lasts for ten days and is performed annually thereafter.

Shruti. "That which is heard"; collectively, early Hindu literature. The Vedas are considered to have been delivered by the gods and heard by the Hindu sages.

Shudra. The lowest of the four castes in India: the toilers and laborers. Many are part of the "scheduled castes" of India: in a schedule appended to the constitution they are given special privileges (as in American affirmative action programs). They are higher than the untouchables, who are without a caste.

Smriti. "That which is remembered"; the later Hindu literature (e.g., the *dharmashastra*)

Sutra. An aphorism or a compendium of aphorisms (e.g., *kamasutra*); literally, that which has been spun or sewn together. Most religious texts are considered *sutras*.

Tantra. A school of Hindu philosophy commonly associated with esoteric sexual practices.

Upanayana. An important Hindu rite of passage into studenthood or apprenticeship, popularly known as the thread ceremony. Literally meaning to go near or toward the teacher.

Upanishads. Ancient Indian metaphysical writings dealing with questions about life and death and considered to be commentaries on the Vedas, which preceded them. There are thirteen major Upanishads (dating from 1000–500 B.C.E.) and over a hundred minor ones.

Vaidya. An Ayurvedic physician.

Vaishya. One of the four castes: traders, bankers, shopkeepers, moneylenders, agriculturalists.

Vedas. The books of knowledge that make up the most ancient Indian religious literature. The *Rig Veda* is the oldest; the others are the *Sam Veda, Yajur Veda,* and *Atharva Veda,* dated 1500–1000 B.C.E.

Yoga. From the root *yuj,* meaning to join, unite, or yoke; the theory and practice of bringing mind and body under control, a form of meditative discipline.

Bibliography

Primary Sources

Aitareya-Aranyaka. Translated by F. Max Muller. In *The Upanishads,* Part 1. New York: Dover, 1962.

The Ananga Ranga of Kalyana Malla. Translated by F. F. Arbuthnot and Richard Burton. New York: Lancer Books, 1964.

The Ananga Ranga: The Hindu Ritual of Love. Translated and edited by Tridibnath Ray. New York: Citadel Press, 1964.

Ashtangahridaya. Text with Gujarati translation by Vijayshankar Dhanshankar Munshi. Ahmedabad: Sastu Sahitya Vardhak Karyalaya, 1983.

Atharvaveda. Translated by Acharya Vaidyanath Shastri. 2 vols. New Delhi: Sarvadeshik Arya Pratinidhi Sabha, 1984.

The Bhagavad Gita. Translated by Franklin Edgerton. New York: Harper and Row, 1964.

The Bhagavadgita in the Mahabharata. Translated by J. A. B. Van Buitenen. Chicago: University of Chicago Press, 1981.

Bhavaprakasha. Gujarati translation by Girijashankar Mayashanker Shastri. 2 vols. Ahmedabad: Sastu Sahitya Vardhak Karyalaya, 1981.

Brihadaranyaka Upanishad. Translated by F. Max Muller. In *The Upanishads,* Part 2. New York: Dover, 1962.

Carakasamhita. Translated by Priyavrat Sharma. 2 vols. Varanasi, India: Chaukhambha Orientalia, 1981–83.

Chandogya Upanishad. Translated by F. Max Muller. In *The Upanishads,* Part 1. New York: Dover, 1962.

Gitagovinda of Jayadeva. Edited and translated as *The Love Song of the Dark Lord* by Barbara Stoler Miller. New York Columbia University Press, 1977.

Hathayogapradipika. Gujarati translation by Vasudev Mahashankar Joshi. Ahmedabad: Sastu Sahitya Vardhak Karyalaya, 1957.

Isa Upanisad. Translated by Swami Gambhirananda, with the commentary of Sankaracarya. In *Eight Upanisads,* vol. 1. Calcutta: Advaita Ashrama, 1977.

Kamasutra of Vatsayana. Translated by Richard F. Burton. New York: E. P. Dutton, 1964.

Katha Upanishad. Translated by F. Max Muller. In *The Upanishads,* Part 2. New York: Dover, 1962.

Kausitaki Upanishad. Translated by F. Max Muller. In *The Upanishads,* Part 1. New York: Dover, 1962.

Kokasastra. Translated by Alex Comfort. New York: Stein and Day, 1965.

The Laws of Manu. Translated by Georg Buhler. New York: Dover, 1969.

The Mahabharata. Translated by J. A. B. Van Buitenen. Chicago: University of Chicago Press, 1973.

Mandukya Upanisad. Translated by Swami Gambhirananda. In *Eight Upanisads,* vol. 2. Calcutta: Advaita Ashrama, 1982.

Patanjali's Yogasutra, with the commentary of Vyasa and the gloss of Vachaspati Misra. Translated by Rama Prasad. New Delhi: Oriental Reprint, 1982.

The Rig Veda: An Anthology. Translated by Wendy Doniger O'Flaherty. Harmondsworth: Penguin Classics, 1981.

Srimad DeviBhagavata Purana. Translated by Swami Vynananda. Sacred Books of the Hindus Series, vol. 26. Allahabad: Bhuvanesvari Ashram, n.d.

Sushrutasamhita. Text with Gujarati translation by Shastri Kalidas Govindji. Ahmedabad: Sastu Sahitya Vardhak Karyalaya, 1973.

Taittiriya Upanishad. Translated by F. Max Muller. *The Upanishads,* Part 2. New York: Dover, 1962.

Valmiki Ramayana. Critical edition by G. H. Bhatt. 7 vols. Baroda, India: Oriental Institute, 1960–75.

Secondary Sources

Allchin, Bridget, and Raymond Allchin. *The Rise of Civilization in India and Pakistan.* Cambridge: Cambridge University Press, 1982.

Basham, A. L. *The Wonder That Was India.* New York: Grove Press, 1959.

Berriedale, Keith A., ed. *The Mythology of All Races,* vol. 6. New York: Cooper Square, 1964.

Campbell, Joseph. *Oriental Mythology: The Masks of God.* New York: Viking Press, 1962.

Carstairs, Morris. "*Hinjra* and *Jiryan:* Two Derivatives of Hindu Attitudes to Sexuality." *British Journal of Medical Psychology* 29 (1956): 128–38.

———. "Medicine and Faith in Rural Rajasthan." In *Health, Culture and Community,* edited by Benjamin D. Paul. New York: Russell Sage, 1955.

Carstairs, Morris, and Ravi Kapur. *The Great Universe of Kota.* Berkeley and Los Angeles: University of California, 1976.

Chandrashekhar, Sripati. *Abortion in a Crowded World: The Problem of Abortion with Special Reference to India.* London: Allen and Unwin, 1974.

Chatterji, Suniti Kumar. "Linguistic Survey of India: Languages and Script." In *The Cultural Heritage of India,* vol. 1, edited by Chatterji et al., 53–75. Calcutta: Ramakrishna Mission, 1958.

Chattopadhyaya, Debiprasad. *Science and Society in Ancient India.* Calcutta: Research India Publications, 1977.

Chaudhari, Nirad. *Hinduism.* New York: Oxford University Press, 1979.

Collins, Alfred, and Prakash Desai. "Selfhood in Context: Some Indian Solutions." In *The Cultural Transition,* edited by Mary White and Susan Pollak, 261–90. Boston: Routledge and Kegan Paul, 1986.

Dandekar, R. N. "Brahminism." In *Sources of Indian Tradition,* edited by William Theodore de Bary et al. New York: Columbia University Press, 1958.

Daniels, Sheryl. "The Tool-box Approach of the Tamil to the Issues of Moral Responsibility and Human Destiny." In *Karma: An Anthropological Inquiry*, edited by Charles Keyes and E. Valentine Daniel, 27–62. Berkeley and Los Angeles: University of California Press, 1983.

Das, Veena. "Paradigms of Body Symbolism: Analysis of Selected Themes in Hindu Culture." In *Indian Religion*, edited by Richard Burghart and Audrey Cantlie, 180–207. London: Curzon Press, 1985.

Dasgupta, Surendranath. *A History of Indian Philosophy*. 5 vols. Delhi: Motilal Banarsidass, 1975.

Desai, Prakash, and George Coelho. "Indian Immigrants in America: Some Cultural Aspects of Psychosocial Adaptation." In *The New Ethnics: Asian Indians in the United States*, edited by Paramatma Saran and Edwin Eames, 363–86. New York: Praeger, 1980.

Dimock, Edward, and Denise Levertov. *In Praise of Krishna: Poems from the Bengali*. Chicago: University of Chicago Press, 1967.

Dumont, Louis. *Homo Hierarchicus*. Chicago: University of Chicago Press, 1980.

Dunn, Fredrick. "Traditional Asian Medicine and Cosmopolitan Medicine as Adaptive Systems." In *Asian Medical Systems*, edited by Charles Leslie, 137–58. Berkeley and Los Angeles: University of California Press, 1976.

Eck, Diana L. *Banaras: City of Light*. Princeton: Princeton University Press, 1983.

Eliade, Mircea. *Patanjali and Yoga*. New York: Schocken Books, 1975.

———. *Yoga: Immortality and Freedom*. Princeton: Princeton University Press, 1970.

Filliozat, Jean. *The Classical Doctrine of Indian Medicine*. Translated by Dev Raj Chanana. Delhi: Munshiram Manoharlal, 1964.

Gandhi, Mohandas. *An Autobiography: The Story of My Experiments with Truth*. Boston: Beacon Press, 1957.

Gonda, Jan. "Indian Religions: An Overview." *Encyclopedia of Religion*, ed. Mircea Eliade, vol. 7. New York: Macmillan, 1987.

Gould, Harold. "The Implications of Technological Change for Folk and Scientific Medicine." *American Anthropologist* 59 (1957): 507–16.

———. "Modern Medicine and Folk Cognition in Rural India." *Human Organization* 24 (1965): 201–8.

Gupta, Mahendranatha. *The Gospel of Sri Ramakrishna*. Translated by Swami Nikhilananda. New York: Ramakrishna-Vivekananda Center, 1942.

Haas, William. *Destiny of the Mind: East and West*. New York: Doubleday, 1956.

Inden, Ronald, and Ralph Nicholas. *Kinship in Bengali Culture*. Chicago: University of Chicago Press, 1977.

India 1985. Compiled and edited by Research and Reference Division, Ministry of Information and Broadcasting. Government of India, 1986.

Jolly, Julius. *Indian Medicine*. Translated by Chintamani Ganesh Kashikar. New Delhi: Munshiram Manoharlal, 1977.

Kakar, Sudhir. *Shamans, Mystics, and Doctors*. New York: Alfred A. Knopf, 1982.

Kane, Pandurang Vaman. *History of Dharmasastra*. 5 vols. Poona: Bhandankar Oriental Research Institute, 1968–77.

Karve, Iravati. "The Indian Social Organization: An Anthropological Study." In *The Cultural Heritage of India*, vol. 2, edited by S. K. De, V. N. Ghoshal, A. D. Pusalkar, and R. C. Hazra. Calcutta: Ramakrishna Mission, 1962.

Knipe, David. "Sapindikarana: The Hindu Rite of Entry into Heaven." In *Religious*

Encounters with Death: Insights from History and Anthropology of Religions, edited by F. E. Reynolds and E. H. Waugh. University Park: University of Pennsylvania Press, 1977.

Kohut, Heinz. *The Search for the Self: Selected Writings of Heinz Kohut, 1950–1978.* Edited by Paul H. Ornstein. 2 vols. New York: International Universities Press, 1978.

Kosambi, Damodar D. *Myth and Reality.* Bombay: Popular Prakashan, 1962.

Leslie, Charles, ed. *Asian Medical Systems.* Berkeley and Los Angeles: University of California Press, 1976.

Lingat, Robert. *The Classical Law of India.* Translated by J. Duncan M. Derrett. Berkeley and Los Angeles: University of California Press, 1973.

McDaniel, June. *"Bhava:* Religious Ecstasy and Madness in Bengal." Ph.D. diss., University of Chicago, 1986.

Marriott, McKim. "Little Communities in an Indigenous Civilization." In *Village India: Studies in the Little Community,* ed. McKim Marriott, 171–222. Chicago: University of Chicago Press, 1969.

———. "The Open Hindu Person and Interpersonal Fluidity." Typescript.

———. "Western Medicine in Northern India." In *Health, Culture and Community,* edited by Benjamin D. Paul, 239–68. New York: Russell Sage, 1955.

Marriott, McKim, and Ronald Inden. *Encyclopedia Britannica,* 15th ed., s.v. "caste system."

———. "Toward an Ethnosociology of South Asian Caste Systems." In *The New Wind: Changing Identities in South Asia,* edited by Kenneth David, 227–38. The Hague: Monton Publishers, 1977.

Miller, Barbara. *The Endangered Sex: Neglect of Female Children in Rural North India.* Ithaca: Cornell University Press, 1981.

Mishra, Rajchatra. *Atharvavedame Sanskritic Tatva* (in Hindi). Allahabad: Punchnad Publishers, 1968.

Murphy, Lois. "Roots of Tolerance and Tensions in Indian Child Development." In *In the Minds of Men,* edited by Gardner Murphy, 46–58. New York: Basic Books, 1953.

Nandy, Ashis. *Alternative Sciences.* New Delhi: Allied Publishers Private Limited, 1980.

———. "An Anti-Secularist Manifesto." *Seminar* 314 (October 1985): 14–24.

———. *At the Edge of Psychology: Essays in Politics and Culture.* Delhi: Oxford University Press, 1980.

Nehru, Jawaharlal. *The Discovery of India.* Delhi: Jawaharlal Nehru Memorial Fund, 1981.

Neki, J. S. "Guru-Chela Relationship: The Possibility of a Therapeutic Paradigm." *American Journal of Orthopsychiatry* 45 (1973): 273–90.

Nichter, Mark. "Negotiation of the Illness Experience: Ayurvedic Therapy and the Psychosocial Dimension of Illness." *Culture, Medicine and Psychiatry* 5 (1981): 5–24.

Obeyesekere, Gananath. "Illness, Culture and Meaning: Some Comments on the Nature of Traditional Medicine." In *Medicine in Chinese Culture,* edited by Arthur Kleinman et al., 253–63. Bethesda, Md.: Fogarty International Center, National Institutes of Health, 1975.

————. "The Rebirth Eschatology and Its Transformation: A Contribution to the Sociology of Early Buddhism." In *Karma and Rebirth in Classical Indian Traditions*, edited by Wendy Doniger O'Flaherty. Berkeley and Los Angeles: University of California Press, 1980.

O'Flaherty, Wendy Doniger. *Hindu Myths*. Harmondsworth: Penguin Books, 1973.

————. *The Origins of Evil in Hindu Mythology*. Berkeley and Los Angeles: University of California Press, 1976.

————. *Women, Androgynes, and Other Mythical Beasts*. Chicago: University of Chicago Press, 1980.

————, ed. *Karma and Rebirth in Classical Indian Traditions*. Berkeley and Los Angeles: University of California Press, 1980.

Organ, Troy. *The Hindu Quest for the Perfection of Man*. Athens: Ohio University Press, 1970.

Otto, Rudolf. *The Idea of the Holy*. Translated by John W. Harvey. New York: Oxford University Press, 1958.

Patel, Raojibhai C. "Personhood in the *Gita*." Paper presented at the Seminar on the Person, University of Chicago, 1978.

Radhakrishnan, Sarvepalli. *Eastern Religion and Western Thought*. London: Oxford University Press, 1940.

Radhakrishnan, Sarvepalli, and Charles A. Moore, eds. *A Sourcebook in Indian Philosophy*. Princeton: Princeton University Press, 1957.

Ramanujan, B. K. "The Indian Family in Transition: Changing Roles and Relationships in the Indian Family: Patterns of Change in the Seventies." *Indian Social Institute* (New Delhi) 2, no. 1 (January–March 1972).

Ray, Priyadaranjan, and Harendra Nath Gupta. *Carakasamhita: A Scientific Synopsis*. New Delhi: National Institute of Sciences of India, 1965.

Rolland, Allan. "Psychoanalytic Perspective on Personality Development in India." *International Review of Psychoanalysis* 7 (1980): 73–88.

Schweitzer, Albert. *Indian Thought and Its Development*. Boston: Beacon Press, 1956.

Sharma, Pandit Shiv, ed. *Realms of Ayurveda*. New Delhi: Arnold-Heinemann, 1979.

Sheth, Dhirubhai L. "Hinduism: An Ecology of Existence." Paper prepared for the United Nations University project on the Perceptions of Desirable Societies in Different Religious and Ethical Systems, Tokyo, 1987.

Somasundaram, O., T. Jayaramakrishnan, and M. Sureshkumar. "Psychiatry in the Siddha (Tamil) System of Medicine." *Indian Journal of Psychological Medicine* 9 (1986): 38–45.

Spear, Percival. *A History of India*, vol. 2. Harmondsworth: Penguin Books, 1978.

Teja, J. S., B. S. Khanna, and T. B. Subramanyam. "Possession States in Indian Patients." *Indian Journal of Psychiatry* 12 (1970): 70–87.

Varma, L. P., D. K. Srivastava, and R. N. Sahay. "Possession Syndrome." *Indian Journal of Psychiatry* 12 (1970): 49–70.

Weiss, Mitchell. "*Carakasamhita* on the Doctrine of *Karma*." In *Karma and Rebirth in Classical Indian Traditions*, edited by Wendy Doniger O'Flaherty, 90–115. Berkeley and Los Angeles: University of California Press, 1980.

Winternitz, Moriz. *History of Indian Literature*. Translated by Subhadra Jha. 3 vols. Delhi: Motilal Banarsidass, 1967.

Zaehner, R. C. *The Bhagavad Gita*. London: Oxford University Press, 1969.
Zimmer, Heinrich. *Myths and Symbols in Indian Art and Civilization*. Edited by Joseph Campbell. Princeton: Princeton University Press, 1972.
———. *The Philosophies of India*. Edited by Joseph Campbell. Princeton: Princeton University Press, 1969.

Index

145

Health/Medicine and the Faith Traditions

HEALTH AND MEDICINE IN THE ANGLICAN TRADITION
David H. Smith

HEALTH AND MEDICINE IN THE CATHOLIC TRADITION
Richard A. McCormick

HEALTH AND MEDICINE IN THE CHRISTIAN SCIENCE TRADITION
Robert Peel

HEALTH AND MEDICINE IN THE HINDU TRADITION
Prakash N. Desai

HEALTH AND MEDICINE IN THE ISLAMIC TRADITION
Fazlur Rahman

HEALTH AND MEDICINE IN THE JEWISH TRADITION
David M. Feldman

HEALTH AND MEDICINE IN THE LUTHERAN TRADITION
Martin E. Marty

HEALTH AND MEDICINE IN THE METHODIST TRADITION
E. Brooks Holifield

HEALTH AND MEDICINE IN THE ORTHODOX TRADITION
Stanley Samuel Harakas

HEALTH AND MEDICINE IN THE REFORMED TRADITION
Kenneth L. Vaux